Health Care Ethics

Arthur H. Parsons, B.Sc., M.D.
and
Patricia Houlihan Parsons,
B.N., M.Sc.

WALL & EMERSON, INC.

nto, Ontario • Middletown, Ohio

Requests for permission to make copies of any part of this work should be sent to: Wall & Emerson, Inc., Six O'Connor Drive, Toronto, Ontario, Canada M4K 2K1

Orders for this book may be directed to either of the following addresses:

For Canada and the rest of the world:	*For the United States:*
Wall & Emerson, Inc.	Wall & Emerson, Inc.
Six O'Connor Drive	3210 S. Main St.
Toronto, Ontario, Canada	P. O. Box 448686
M4K 2K1	Middletown, Ohio 45044-8686

By telephone or facsimile (for both addresses):

Telephone: (416) 467-8685
Fax: (416) 696-2460

Canadian Cataloguing in Publication Data

Parsons, Arthur H. (Arthur Hedley), 1943-

  Health care ethics

Includes index.
ISBN 1-895131-08-1

1. Medical ethics. I. Parsons, Patricia Houlihan.
II. Title.

R724.P37 1992   174'.2   C92-093366-1

ISBN 1-895131-08-1
Printed in the United States by Haddon Craftsmen.

 1 2 3 4 5   95 94 93 92

Photograph of authors on back cover by Garey Pridham.

Contents

List of Figures

Introduction

Health care ethics is truly the point at which the art of medicine, our ability to be humane and compassionate, meets the science of medicine, as manifested in clinical health care by medical technology and modern pharmacology. The purpose of this book is to provide a starting point from which both students and practitioners in a variety of health disciplines may develop a frame of reference for bringing humanity into their delivery of modern health care. Whether the health care provider is a nurse practitioner, a dentist, a physiotherapist, a physician, or any other, whenever there are decisions of right or wrong, good or bad to be made, that health care worker is at the interface between the patient and the decision. When the interface between technology and humanity is also involved, the dilemmas are even more complex.

The amazing advances in technology that have saved so many lives have also given rise to serious ethical problems, such as how to fairly distribute increasingly scarce resources, maintain confidentiality, support patient autonomy, define death and life, and the list goes on and on. We argue that as a result of the changes in the delivery of health care and the resources available, we need to move away from the strictly individual patient-centered ethics that has been the cornerstone of our relationships with patients, and consider the broader context of the common good and our responsibilities to society as a whole.

After years of practice in family medicine, general and critical care nursing, medical communications and teaching health care ethics, we have concluded that a text in health care ethics should be immediately relevant to the real world of health care delivery, clear in its discussions, and of practical use to the health care professional—in other words, "user-friendly," which we intend this book to be.

The text is organized into three sections. The first introduces some of the principles that underlie the current issues which are then presented in section two. Part three deals with issues that grow out of our professional relationships and consultations. The concept of interprofessional etiquette may not seem, at first glance, to be of ethical importance or interest, but the increasingly multidisciplinary nature of health care delivery makes it a vital issue for the future, and since it is our intent to be useful to a variety of disciplines, this aspect of professional behavior is very important. Finally, we examine the emerging role of a new health team member, the medical ethicist. For those who require a more substantial dose of academia, we provide carefully selected recommended readings for each topic discussed and a glossary of ethical terms.

We believe that physicians, nurses, and other allied health professionals need to be aware of one other important issue—the image of health care and health care ethics projected by the popular media, which provides a large proportion of health care information for vast numbers of North Americans and has had a significant impact in creating consumer demands in health care. Thus, we refer to and also recommend a number of information sources outside the traditional professional and academic literature. Since ethics is becoming an issue of particular importance in public policy determination, the lay literature cannot be ignored.

This book, however, is not a cookbook, nor do we believe that there are black-and-white answers. Several years ago, one of us was involved in teaching health care ethics to first-year student nurses. After class one day, a young student came up and said, "Every day I come into your ethics classes and I think I am clear about how I feel about the issues." (This was a rather frightening statement coming from a nineteen-year-old, less than six months into her nursing education!) She continued, "And every time I leave class, I'm more confused than when I went in." Although it is doubtful that she meant it as a compliment, it was taken as such, because a primary goal in teaching health care ethics to neophyte practitioners should be to make them think about all of the issues in their full complexity so that, as they come to know more about the science of their field, they will be better able to see how they can be involved in humane decision making.

Thus, it is our objective to give you, in a practical way, some basic information about the underlying principles of health care ethics and to make you think about your own values and how they fit with what is expected of you in your role as a caregiver.

Arthur H. Parsons, B.Sc., M.D.
Patricia Houlihan Parsons, B.N., M.Sc.

January 1992

Part I

The Context

1

Art Meets Science: Why Study Ethics Anyway?

In this chapter:

- ■ Everyday ethical dilemmas

- ■ Current social trends that create and/or affect these dilemmas

- ■ A definition of ethics

- ■ Approaches to ethical decision making
  - Rule ethics
  - Situational ethics
- ■ Principles of medical ethics
  - Sanctity of life
  - Beneficence/non-maleficence
  - Personal autonomy
  - Justice

Man is an animal with primary instincts of survival. Consequently, his ingenuity has developed first and his soul second. Thus the progress of science is far ahead of man's ethical behavior.

From *My Autobiography*, 1964 by Sir Charles
Spencer Chaplin (better known as Charlie)

It was two minutes past eight a.m. when Dr. Brian Moral pulled into the doctor's parking lot and eased his BMW into the last available space. The parking problems at St. Swithin's Hospital were legion, and he breathed a sigh of relief that he would not have to park illegally, yet again, as he made rounds to see three obstetrical patients and one elderly lady whose daughter had made him promise to get in to see her this morning.

A very busy family doctor with a full day ahead of him, he took a minute to make a few notes in his date book before getting out of the car. While he was scribbling he heard a noise behind the car and glanced in the rearview mirror just in time to see Dr. Skittish, an esteemed St. Swithin's surgeon, sideswipe a sleek, new Jaguar. Dr. Skittish got out, checked the scratch which was plainly visible, glanced furtively around, got back into his car and drove away. It was plain that he hadn't seen Dr. Moral sitting in his car.

Dr. Moral shook his head and snorted. He momentarily considered reporting what he had just witnessed to the hospital traffic control officer at the front desk, but decided simply to mention it to Dr. Skittish the next time their paths crossed, which he fervently hoped would not be too soon.

He double-checked on his patients' room numbers with the receptionist at the front desk and hurried to the bank of elevators where a few people were waiting. He stepped into the elevator and pressed the button for the eighth floor where he would look in on his elderly patient first.

The elevator stopped at the second floor where the intensive care units were located, and an intern and a respiratory technologist got on. It was apparent from their conversation that they had just come from an unsuccessful cardiac arrest.

"You're getting pretty good at that intubation stuff," the technologist said to the intern.

"Nothing to it. When you can't bring them back, you get to practice a few times. They call a code on so many old geezers around here, we get lots of practice." They both laughed.

Dr. Moral and the other people on the elevator, who appeared to be day surgery patients heading to the operating room, moved to the back of the elevator as a group of doctors and nurses, evidently in the middle of rounds, got on, still deep in conversation.

"Who are we seeing next?" asked the older doctor, who appeared to be the clinician conducting the rounds.

One of the nurses looked at the clipboard in her hand. "It's Judith Evans." They all groaned and looked at each other.

"Can we skip her today?" asked one of the residents.

The older doctor cleared his throat, looked disapprovingly at the resident and continued, "Yes, yes, a difficult situation indeed. Consider, if you will, ladies and gentlemen, a young woman struck down with kidney disease in the prime of her life, not responding well to dialysis…"

"She'd respond well if she'd take her medication and follow her diet," continued the resident. "I'm beginning to think people like her—people who won't even do what we tell them—should fall in line behind others…"

Dr. Moral didn't hear any more of this elevator conversation as they had reached his floor. One of the other occupants also disembarked, stone-faced.

As Dr. Moral headed toward the nursing station of the medical floor where his elderly patient was located, he passed several rooms occupied by aging patients. Most, he noted to himself, were restrained.

He was thumbing through the patient's chart just as the head nurse and one of the senior internists came around the corner.

"Doctor," the nurse was saying, "if you have a complaint about the nurses I would appreciate if in future you would come to me, so that I can deal with the situation. What was the name of the nurse who made you so angry?"

The doctor looked at her over the tops of his half glasses. "They have names?"

Dr. Moral stifled a smile. Just then, two student nurses and a nursing instructor Dr. Moral recognized as a former staff nurse came out of the adjoining conference room.

"She does have the right to refuse to have you look after her," the instructor was saying to an obviously distraught student.

"She's only refusing because I'm black and you know it. It's not her right."

As they went down the hall, Dr. Moral followed them as far as his patient's room where he had a quick visit and then headed upstairs to the obstetrical floor, where the situation was generally happier and calmer. The nursing station was also filled with people on early morning rounds, but rounds here always included not only the usual doctors and nurses, but also the patient education coordinator, a social worker, and sometimes a pharmacist, physiotherapist, or respiratory technologist if the patients had any other medically related problems. Here, they truly believed in the team approach and practised what they preached.

"I think we should be doing everything we can to encourage her to maintain the pregnancy so that the baby can be used as an organ donor," said one of the nurses.

"I'm not even sure I like what they've been doing with these anencephalic newborns," said another.

"I can tell you I wouldn't want to be walking around knowing I was carrying a deformed baby. Just imagine what it would do to your psyche. It wouldn't matter to me one bit that someone else's kid just might, and I stress *might*, benefit. I'd be a basket case for the rest of my life."

Dr. Moral quickly reviewed the charts of his new mothers and was grateful to see that they all had had normal deliveries, with normal outcomes. Just before seeing them, his next stop would be the nursery.

"Good morning, Dr. Moral," the charge nurse greeted him. "Are you going to do the circumcision on Baby Jones? Dr. Fence couldn't talk her out of it." Dr. Fence was one of his partners and this would not be the first time Dr. Moral had done a circumcision on one of his patients. Dr. Fence believed them to be unnecessary surgery and refused to do them anymore.

As he drove back across town, Dr. Moral was grateful that he didn't meet any ethical dilemmas in his daily practice!

There is no question that, despite his perception, Dr. B. Moral was exposed to a significant number of ethical conundra before his working day had really even begun. And those problems were broad, general ones that hinge on general principles and did not even begin to take into account the individual concerns of the patients involved. Perhaps even more alarming, though, is the fact that Dr. Moral believes that he does not face ethical dilemmas in his daily practice. This is a dangerous misapprehension for any health professional.

Let's examine some of the questions raised by Dr. Moral's experience.

- Is it ever appropriate for health professionals to discuss patients on elevators, or within the confines of the hospital, even when it saves them precious time so that they can see more patients?
- Is the use of recently deceased patients to teach health professionals how to do procedures ever justified? Would it be justifiable never to use them?

- Should non-compliant patients have their access to care restricted to make way for the more compliant?
- How do you define what is acceptable in the provision of a sufficiently high level of dignity for our elderly patients?
- What role does respect play in interprofessional relationships?
- Do patients have the right to refuse to be treated by individual health professionals, regardless of the reason?
- To what extent do the personal values of the health care provider affect moral decisions made for patients?
- Can a health professional refuse to treat a patient because he or she does not agree with the patient's decision? Under what circumstances can he or she refuse?

Ethics is a subject of much interest today. In many areas, such as politics, business, the law, etc., the ethical problems that abound are receiving much exposure and serious concern. And, in spite of the fact that ethics has concerned health care providers for centuries, the current concern, as evidenced by a growing body of literature on the subject, is more pressing than ever. Is this because our generation is more sensitive than health care workers of the past? A more likely explanation is that we are "frightened by our ability to influence decisions regarding life and death yet, at the same time, unable to fix guidelines for compassion and justice" (Levine, 1977, p. 845). Maybe it's time to take a second look at Charlie Chaplin's observation, made at the beginning of this chapter. For all our high-tech machinery and our arsenal of drugs, perhaps we need to recognize that it just may be true that scientific progress is, indeed, outdistancing our ethical behavior.

Current Social Trends

Medical Advances

Edward Shorter has described the century that is now drawing to a close as the "health century" (Shorter, 1987) because of the incredible medical advances made since 1900. Before that time health care workers could provide care, but *they could not cure disease*. And that change, from care to cure, perhaps more than anything else, has fundamentally changed the practice of medicine and led to the tremendous current concern for ethics. When the most a doctor had to offer a child dying of kidney failure was comfort measures and a strong hand to hold, the dilemma of who should receive the available kidney for transplant never arose. Health care professionals must now give more than a passing thought to concerns other than simply the care of their patients.

Rise of Consumerism

Other developments have led to an increased need to address ethics in health care. One of these is the rise of consumerism. In 1962, President John F. Kennedy declared that every consumer has four basic rights:

- the right to be informed;
- the right to safety;
- the right to choose;
- the right to be heard (Newsom, Scott and Turk, 1989).

The delineation of these rights may appear to be a simple reiteration of the basic rights of every human being. However, until the early twentieth century, big business, in the persons of such industrialists as Rockefeller and Vanderbilt, had such power and control that they could truly afford their well-known "public be damned" attitude. Only after a few journalists brought the appalling treatment of workers to public attention did business begin responding to labor's demands for improved working conditions and wages. This turn of events could be viewed as paving the way for what became the grass roots consumer movement that had its beginnings in the 1950s. Kennedy's public acknowledgement of those rights lent strength and credibility to a movement that would have an irreversible impact on every aspect of the provision of consumer goods and services, one of which is health care.

Consumer activism gained momentum as medical technology entered a period of rapid growth. This technological progress turned health care into a consumable product like any other and marked the beginning of changes in traditional relationships with patients. For example, a patient who is more informed about the alternative methods for treating any number of conditions is less likely to accept at face value what a health provider says, adding a different and initially unpleasant dimension to the exchange.

Before the concept of consumer rights was recognized by health care workers, only the exhortation to be committed to patient safety was taken seriously. The idea that patients should be informed so as to freely exercise their right to choose was unheard of at the beginning of this century. Thus, without a doubt, the ideas and effects of the consumer movement spilled over into the delivery of health care across North America.

Increase in Professional Disciplines

Another twentieth century development has been the proliferation of disciplines within the health care system. At the turn of the century, the physician and the nurse were the cornerstones of health care delivery. By the early 1980s, more than 5.1 million Americans were employed in 700 different occupational fields in health care. Of these, only 600,000 were medical practitioners, while over 3 million were nurses (Consumer Guide, 1982).

This diversification of backgrounds in health care delivery has had and continues to have a number of effects on both relationships with patients and other health professionals. First, consumers are unsure of the qualifications of those providing care. When a patient enters the hospital, he or she encounters a wide variety of individuals, with varying responsibilities, even within the same discipline. The patient may be involved with head nurses, nursing supervisors, student nurses, staff nurses, practical nurses, nurses' aides, nurse practitioners, infection control nurses, to mention only a few in one field alone. Patients who are not already familiar with this diversity must find their situation confusing and fragmented. In addition, patients are often in a quandary as to what kind of practitioner ought to be giving them care. For example, a patient with low back pain might find it difficult to decide if that condition should be treated by a nurse practitioner, a chiropractor, a physiotherapist, an orthopedic surgeon, or the family doctor.

The second effect of this proliferation of health care disciplines is the development and growth of a competitive marketplace mentality. The poor patient who cannot decide about care for low back pain will probably encounter different points of view on optimum treatment, depending on which kind of professional is first consulted. The patient becomes a football to be fought over and passed around.

The final effect, a consequence of this growing marketplace mentality, is increasing numbers of jurisdictional disputes. As each discipline attempts to carve out recognized roles, some jurisdictional boundaries become less distinct. Interprofessional squabbling is an increasingly common phenomenon, and the patient is often caught in the middle.

Budgetary Restraints

No discussion of health care in the 1990s would be complete without mentioning the fiscal restraints that have tightened purse strings and had serious effects on both public and private health care in North America. In 1989, for example, health care spending in the US reached an all-time high of $604 billion dollars, which represents about $2400 spent on every man, woman, and child in the country. In Canada, where the health care delivery system is publicly funded, health care now costs the government in the vicinity of $46 billion every year (Rachlis, 1989). In the foreseeable future the situation will only worsen as health costs increase, forcing health professionals on every level to face dilemmas caused by scarcity of health care resources. Rationing, or the restriction of services, has become a dirty word in medical circles, but the hard economic realities felt at both the system and the patient level demand some kind of solution.

Increasing Numbers of Elderly Patients

Our population is swiftly aging. The much publicized phenomenon of the greying of America has direct consequences for the delivery of health care services. Currently, about 12% of the American population is over the age of 65. At the present rate of growth, population projections indicate that by the year 2230 over 20%, or possibly even as high as 27%, of Americans will be counted among the aged. For practical purposes we need to look at these numbers from a different perspective. In early 1990, to herald the new decade, *Newsweek* carried a special edition about the family in the 21st century. In the article entitled "The Geezer Boom," statistics from the US Census Bureau indicated that by the year 2005 there will be 100 middle-aged people for every 114 people over the age of 65, and by 2025, for every 100 middle-aged Americans, there will be 253 seniors (Beck, 1990).

It is certain that we are going to face a vastly increased economic burden since a huge proportion of health care dollars is spent to provide care for the elderly. Perhaps of even more concern is the question of how we are going to be able to deal with the staggering medical needs of this population while still providing for them a modicum of dignity.

Role of the Media

Developments and issues in medicine and health care have become steady front-page news. Burkett (1986) contends that "nowhere else are threads of scientific enterprise more tangled with economic, political, personality, and social values than in medicine and health care" (p. 100); this is the reason why these stories play so well in the media.

Over the past two decades, the media's response to and coverage of dramatic medical developments has made them important sources of health information for increasing numbers of North Americans. Unfortunately, this development does not always work to the benefit of the patient or the health care worker. The media has its own agenda and makes its own decisions about what is and what is not newsworthy; journalists and medical scientists often disagree about what the public ought to be told and when.

Consumers are particularly vulnerable to media-generated hype. With little ability to differentiate between the truly useful medical breakthrough with immediate consequences for health care delivery, and those media-generated stories that, while based on facts, have little to offer in the foreseeable future, the poor patient either doesn't know what to believe or believes it all. In late 1991, for example, the Canadian press carried a story about a group of scientists from Edmonton, Alberta, employees of a research firm, who are working on a new cancer treatment which involves the use of antibodies tagged with radiation. Directly under the headline

Summary of Social Trends Affecting Health Care Delivery

- The rise of consumerism in society

- The proliferation of allied health disciplines

- The escalating costs of health care

- The aging population in North America

- The role of the mass media

- Technological advances

Figure 1.1.

was a very large and prominent quotation from one of the scientists: "It's like a magic bullet. You're targeting the radiation right at the tumor."

Consider the position of the patient with cancer—the words "magic bullet" are likely to produce a wave of hope. Then consider the position of the reporter writing the story—this highly dramatic and quotable phrase is a gift that cannot be refused. Finally, consider the position of the patient's family doctor when the patient excitedly arrives in the office with this story. If up-to-date with current medical news, the doctor must now explain to the disappointed patient that the article actually went on to say that the firm was *set to begin developing a new treatment based on laboratory research.*

Thus, widespread media attention is also changing the traditional relationship between the physician or other health care worker and the patient. The media is a new player in the health care delivery arena, and a powerful one that cannot be ignored.

We now come back to where we began. The major modern development responsible for pushing ethical concerns to the forefront is the rapid pace of technological advances in medicine. The discoveries that have saved hundreds of thousands of lives have ushered in the era of high-tech medicine. This medicine is glamorous, it is high-profile, but it is available and necessary for only a relatively few people. New medical technologies have brought people back from the dead, have given us new ways of making babies, have allowed us to replace diseased body parts, and have presented every health professional with ethical dilemmas of enormous proportions because, as Charlie Chaplin pointed out to us, science is, indeed, far ahead of our ethical behavior.

What Is Ethics, Anyway?

It should now be fairly clear that ethics is a concern that is not going to go away. So, do you really know what ethics is? There are as many definitions of ethics as there are individuals who have written on the subject. While all of the definitions have a number of things in common, all have slightly different nuances of meaning. In this book, we are concerned with the ethics of health care. Here is our definition:

> *Health care ethics is the application of human values of right or wrong to making meaningful moral choices in health care delivery.*

The definition can be broken down into a number of components:

- Ethics itself is a theoretical discipline within philosophy, intended to distinguish good from bad. Health care ethics, however, is the practical application of ethical principles to health care situations. Knowledge of all the ethical theories and theorists in the world will not help the nurse or doctor or technician decide what he/she ought to do if there is no practical application.
- Some human values of good and bad have endured over time, and some have changed with changes in society. Moreover, each fledgling health care professional brings to the study of science an already established personal value system. Learning about ethics in medical, nursing, or allied health schools has not been shown to change those basic values with which we thus must learn to work.
- Health care ethics is concerned with how to make meaningful choices when faced with dilemmas. Dilemmas are special problems which seem either to have no satisfactory solution or to present a choice between equally undesirable alternatives (Aroskar, 1980). In these difficult situations choices must be made by those who choose to work in health care.

Approaches to Decision Making in Ethics

If only we always knew intuitively how to do the right thing! Unfortunately, as far as we know the human genetic structure does not include the capacity to make the right moral decision in situations encountered in our daily practice. As a result, we face many uncertainties in our struggle to apply health science ethics. These uncertainties, coupled with the effort to manage our own primal feelings and the emotions triggered by the things that we witness every day, often lead to the development of an artificial distance between ourselves and our patients (Fox, 1990) and a disinclination to face ethical dilemmas. The case of Dr. Moral and his observations and reactions at the beginning of this chapter may seem exaggerated, but that hypothetical scenario is drawn from actual scenes witnessed by these authors at one time or another. Problematic situations do exist; difficult choices must be made. How, then, can we be assisted in making ethical decisions?

There are many ways of constructing a framework for ethical decision making; the literature on the subject presents many theories on which these frameworks are based. A framework of this nature can only be effective, though, if it is consistent and practical, and if those who are using it understand it.

Rule Ethics

There are two basic ways of thinking about the solution to an ethical problem. The first approach has been called *rule ethics*. The rules to be followed are set down by an outside source (such as organized religion) or are agreed upon by a group (such as the Canadian or American Medical Association) and are codified. These rules are considered to be fundamental and irrevocable and based on universal ethical principles. They are then used as the basis for making decisions in ethical dilemmas. The application of consistent ethical principles under defined conditions does have a certain appeal to those who do not feel qualified to make difficult decisions nor are comfortable with changing the application of the rules to fit the situation. For example, a health care worker who believes in the strict application of the principle that upholds the sanctity of life will have difficulty understanding the humanity that might be involved in disconnecting the respirator of a patient in irreversible coma. Rigid application of this so-called rule would absolve this worker of ever having to make a decision; it also would remove any degree of flexibility in the assessment of an individual patient's situation. In addition, this approach does not allow for differences that may exist between the rules and the personal value system of the individual decision-maker.

Situational Ethics

The second basic approach to ethical decision making has been termed *situational ethics*. In this approach, the decision-making process includes consideration of the circumstances of the situation, as well as fundamental ethical principles. This allows the decision-maker to apply those principles that seem appropriate in the particular circumstances. For example, abortion can be deemed wrong under one set of circumstances (to select the sex of offspring), yet considered right under others (to end pregnancy due to incest). Using this approach, some people choose to evaluate the outcomes of the decision (a utilitarian ethic) to determine if the ends justify the means. The alternative with the greatest social benefit is chosen after an analysis of the social benefits and costs of each. For example, consider the dilemma faced by a heart transplant team when a heart of a particular blood group becomes

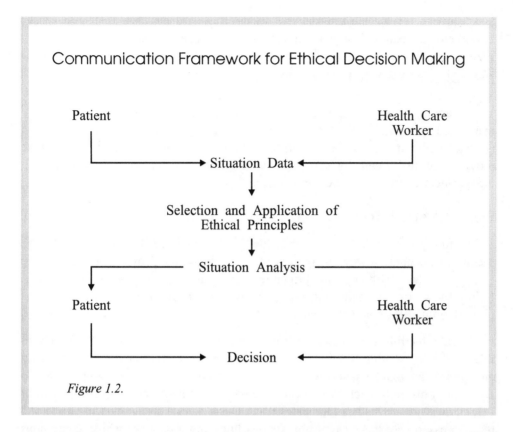

Figure 1.2.

available. If there are two patients who are equivalent from a medical point of view, then how is the decision made about who will receive this organ? If the team were to apply the principle of greatest social benefit, they would be more likely to select for transplant the father of three children than the unemployed drifter.

The use of situational ethics to solve dilemmas has recently become more popular as practitioners find it more and more difficult to apply the so-called ethical laws equally to everyone in every unique set of circumstances. Unfortunately, because patients do not usually have the depth of understanding that health team members do, or ought to, it can be very difficult for them to see how and why the rules do not appear to be applied in the same way all the time. Without excellent communication between the health care providers and patients, those who are directly affected by the decisions may feel that they are not being treated fairly.

There is no one right way to approach the solution of ethical dilemmas in health care. Ideally, though, the patient ought to be a partner with the health care worker, who needs to use both ethical principles and an independent analysis of the situation to come to a decision. Figure 1.2 indicates the flow of information and thought that ought to take place when health care workers face ethical problems and seek solutions. In light of the current societal trends, it should be clear that with proper information the patient is now a full partner in the process.

Principles of Ethics

You are probably wondering by now what are these ethical principles that are mentioned again and again. A principle, of course, is a general truth or a law which is basic to other truths. There are four fundamental principles which have guided the provision of health care for centuries. Although easy to understand on their own, these principles are far more complicated in their application.

Sanctity of Life

The first principle is the concept of the sanctity of life. Life is considered to be precious and should always be preserved; accordingly, the provision of health care is a sacred trust. Although this principle sounds simple, self-evident, and easy to follow and carry out, modern technology has made its application extremely complex. Defining life and death are not easy tasks today.

Consider the following scenario. You are a nurse in the emergency department of a large, urban teaching hospital. You have just spent the past several hours giving emergency care to a teenaged boy who has sustained a head injury from the head-on collision of his motorcycle with a car. He is on a ventilator and the cardiac monitor ticking away above his head indicates that he is in normal sinus rhythm with strong blood pressure. He has several intravenous lines and a catheter whose continuous clear drainage indicates normal kidney function. Unfortunately, he has fixed and dilated pupils with no brain-stem reflexes, and timed removal from the ventilator indicates that he is unable to breathe independently. The EEG technician has just completed the first of two planned EEG's, and the results indicate brain death. You and the resident have just given the family the bad news. They look at him lying on the stretcher and tell you they don't believe he is dead. Unfortunately, today's methods of determining life and death are much harder to understand than they were at the turn of the century.

Beneficence and Non-Maleficence

The second principle is that of *doing good and doing no harm* (beneficence and non-maleficence respectively). This principle is relatively self-explanatory—it is the duty of the health care provider to do the best for the patient under the circumstances and not to harm the patient. Yet, the obligation to follow this rule constantly creates dilemmas in health care delivery, and, once again, modern technology is the main culprit. With advances in diagnostic and surgical procedures and the tremendous increase in the number and efficacy of drugs available to treat every manner of illness, each time a treatment, test, or drug is ordered and carried out, all involved must consider the benefits versus the risks to the patient. For example, when a severely terminally ill cancer patient develops pneumonia, the health care team must decide whether or not to treat. Will the treatment only prolong the agony and therefore do harm to the patient, or will the treatment make the patient more comfortable and therefore be of benefit? Before the advent of antibiotics, this question, of course, would never have arisen.

Individual Autonomy

The third basic ethical principle in health care is one that has become steadily more important over time. This is the concept of personal liberty or, as the ethicists put it, *autonomy*. When a health care worker applies this principle to the solution of an ethical dilemma, he/she is considering the fact that patients have the right to make their own decisions and should be provided with the information necessary to do so. The patient becomes a full partner in the provision of health care.

At the other end of the continuum from patient autonomy is the concept of paternalism, which allows the health care system and all its players to treat the patient like a child who is unable to make proper decisions. Consider the patient with a half dozen seriously decayed teeth sitting in the dentist's chair. The dentist knows that the teeth can be saved but that this will require endodontic treatment (root canal therapy). The patient's response is to request that the dentist simply extract the offending teeth. Knowing that this is not optimum dental care, the dentist refuses. This belief that the "doctor knows best" has led to many an ethical problem.

Justice

Finally, guiding the decisions of the health care worker is the concept of *justice*. Adherence to this principle requires us to treat every patient as equal and provide equivalent treatment for everyone with the same problem. This principle can be sorely tested in situations where there simply is not enough to go around. We present the practical implications of this in a later chapter.

Summary

By now you will realize that simply graduating from a recognized school of medicine, nursing, physiotherapy, or any other health profession does not guarantee ethical competence. Both you and your patient know this. However, what makes you tick as a person is probably more important in the long run than the number of medical ethics courses you take or the number of ethical principles that you remember. You bring to each clinical encounter your own set of values and morals, most of which will stay with you throughout your life. Finally, it is not enough simply to have good intentions; ethical decisions in health care must be based on competence in both the clinical components of your field and the philosophical/compassionate component of your work. This is truly when art meets science.

In summary, to provide ethical care the health care practitioner needs:

- the ability to know when an ethical problem exists;
- the ability to analyze conflicting rights and obligations;
- a workable framework for decision making;
- a commitment to include the patient in the care;
- the ability to recognize when his/her personal values come into conflict with those of the patient.

Questions for Discussion and/or Review

1. Choose any question on pages 5-6 and state or write your position. On which ethical principle(s) do you base your response?

2. Choose any two problems that Dr. Moral encountered and discuss which ethical principles were ignored. How could these problems have been better handled?

3. Discuss any ethical problems you have encountered in your health care experience. Were you able to recognize them as ethical problems when first encountered?

4. Choose any dilemma raised in this chapter. How would the application of rule ethics assist you in making a decision? Situational ethics?

Recommended Reading

Aroskar, Mila A. "Anatomy of an Ethical Dilemma," *American Journal of Nursing*, 80 (April, 1980), 658–660.

Callahan, Daniel. "Shattuck Lecture: Contemporary Biomedical Ethics," *New England Journal of Medicine*, 302 (May 29, 1980), 1228–1233.

Fowler, Marsha. "Bioethics Research in Nursing and Medicine," *Heart-Lung*, 19 (March, 1990), 206–207.

Holmes, Oliver Wendell. "Practical Ethics of the Physician," *Humane Medicine*, 4 (November, 1988), 129–130. (An address to the medical graduates of Harvard University at the annual commencement, March 10, 1858.)

Veatch, Robert M. "Hospital Pharmacy: What is Ethical?" *American Journal of Hospital Pharmacy*, 46 (January, 1989), 109–115.

2

Our Contract with Society

In this chapter:

■ Codes of ethics

■ Problems with codes of ethics

- Lack of concreteness

- Multiple interpretations

- Contradictions and conflicts

- Outdated focus

■ Models of interprofessional care

- Benevolent autocrat model

- Professional independence model

- Health squad model

*I swear by Apollo Physician and Aesculapius and Hygieia and Panaceia
and all the gods and goddesses, making them my witnesses, that I will
fulfil this oath and this covenant according to my ability and judgement.*

Preamble to the Hippocratic Oath, 4th century B.C.

When an individual chooses a career in the health professions, that person enters into a contract with society. This has been so for thousands of years, and for all that time, those involved in provision of health care have attempted to develop a code of principles to guide them in making decisions. These decisions are becoming more complex with each passing year; every time a new technological innovation appears, new and difficult questions about how to do the right thing arise.

The Hippocratic Oath and Codes of Ethics

In the fourth century B.C. the medical profession took upon itself the task of adopting an oath that would explain to each other and to those outside the profession its ideals of how medicine ought to be practised. That oath, attributed to Hippocrates, is what we now know as the Hippocratic Oath (presented in its entirety in the appendices), and its name, at least, is familiar to many members of the general public, who believe that doctors all take this oath and that it is sacred to them. This is not true; nor would taking the oath provide assurance to the health care consumer as to the ethical level of care that will be offered by those who swear. This holds true for the Florence Nightingale pledge for nurses or any other oath that might be taken by a graduating health professional.

A study of 300 physicians revealed that only 32% had even taken the oath at graduation from medical school and that a similar number never read their professional code of ethics (Balkos, 1983)! In addition, the Hippocratic Oath itself has a major loophole. Note that in the preamble it indicates that the duties that follow are to be carried out *"according to my ability and judgement."* By introducing a subjective qualification to the oath, the physician is given a way out of adhering strictly to the requirements. And he, presumably, is the first judge of his ability and judgment.

The codes of ethics of both the American and the Canadian Medical Associations were developed just after the middle of the nineteenth century and were based on the work of the British Medical Association. Revised on several occasions to keep up with the times, these codes are best viewed as the formal contracts of North American medicine with society. Similar codes have been established by other health professions as well. The American Nurses' Association has had a code of ethics since 1950 and the Canadian Nurses' Association since 1980.

One of the main purposes of codes of ethics for the practitioner is that, at least to some extent, they help define the basic nature of the relationship that we, as health care providers, ought to have with our patients, with each other, and with society. Principles that remind us to consider first the well-being of the patient, honor our professions, recognize our limitations (CMA, 1990), as well as not reveal patient confidences, and safeguard the public from colleagues known to lack professional or moral competence (AMA, 1990), are beneficial in helping us deal with our patients and co-workers. Caution, however, is absolutely necessary when attempting to use these codes as formal laws guiding daily ethical practice.

Problems in Using Codes

Codes of ethics are not recipes to solve ethical dilemmas. The application of any part of any code of professional ethics to the solution of real predicaments can only be viewed as one of the steps in the ethical decision-making process. Problems arising in the application of these guidelines include a lack of concreteness, multiple interpretations, and conflicting demands placed on the health care worker.

Lack of Concreteness

One of the main problems with codes of ethics, of which all practitioners need to be aware, is that they are abstract, not concrete, and therefore fail to deal specifically with controversial issues (Sawyer, 1989). In attempting to use codes of ethics for guidance, the health professional will not find precise answers. While this may be viewed as a weakness from the perspective of the individual searching for guidelines, the more definite a set of guidelines, the more cumbersome it becomes, and indeed, the more frequently it needs to be updated. For instance, in today's fast-paced world of technology, to be comprehensive a modern code of ethics would have to provide distinct and detailed guidelines for such issues as abortion, euthanasia, allocation of resources in many areas, reproductive technology, AIDS testing, consent of incompetent individuals, brain death, surrogate motherhood, and on and on. The list would be endless and inevitably incomplete.

Instead, the codes provide general direction and cannot be relied upon as a rulebook with actual solutions to ethical dilemmas. Health professionals, who are used to dealing with the scientific basis of medicine and health care, may find this of particular concern when looking for hard answers to real questions.

Multiple Interpretations and Conflicts

In addition to their lack of concreteness, sections of the codes, because they are open to interpretation, can be viewed as contradictory. For example, Article 6 of the Canadian Medical Association's code of ethics (1990) states that the physician will "keep in confidence information derived from a patient or from a colleague regarding that patient" unless the patient gives permission to break that confidence or the law requires it. Yet, Article 47 of the same code indicates that the physician "will accept a share of the profession's responsibility to society in matters relating to the health and safety of the public." How, then, does this code assist the doctor in dealing with a situation of, for example, the discovery of a commercial airline pilot with an alcohol problem, a drug problem, epilepsy? Does the employer have a right to know about it? Does the physician have the obligation to ensure that potential passengers of the pilot are aware of the risks? That code of ethics will be of little help to the doctor in dealing with this conundrum. And this is only one example of the many problems that cannot be solved by relying on a rulebook solution.

Outdated Focus

The Hippocratic tradition of health care ethics encouraged the belief that our only concern should be for the individual, and that our contract is strictly with the individual patient. Current societal changes, which are now being reflected in most of the codes, are forcing us to realize that, like it or not, our contract is not only with the individual patient, but also with society in general. This is probably the newest of the principles that ought to guide our decisions in ethical health care.

> While once the critical controversies in medical ethics dealt with personal problems faced by patients or health professionals, the ethics of medicine must now be essentially social. The central and controversial issues involve complex social, political and economic relationships and the increasing lay involvement in medical-ethical decision-making. (Veatch, 1984, p. 2296)

Models of Interprofessional Care

Just as the number of critical ethical problems of health care has grown enormously in the recent past, and continues to do so, so too have the issues surrounding the question of what member of the health team is ultimately responsible for the care of the patient. The recent proliferation of disciplines in health care delivery has made it necessary for us to have some guidelines about how we should relate to one another. Without these guidelines, we create new areas of controversy that will, and already do, contribute to even more ethical dilemmas and interfere with the provision of care.

We will now consider three basic models of interprofessional care.

The Benevolent Autocrat Model

This is probably the oldest and most traditional way of organizing the multidisciplinary group of health care workers that grows larger with each passing year. In this model of interprofessional relationships, one profession takes charge. Traditionally, this was the medical profession—the doctor was clearly in command. Of course, this leadership role was accompanied by the doctor's acceptance of the responsibility and accountability for any decisions made. The problem with this model is that it is not based upon, and does not presume, any mutual respect among the members of the health care group or provide for the inclusion of the patient in the decision-making process.

The Professional Independence Model

In this model the disciplines are independent of one another. They go about their assigned tasks with little concern for other health care workers, never interfering, rarely assisting. The patient receives specialized input from each discipline. This is a particularly vexing way of relating to other health care disciplines, especially when the problems are ethical in nature. Each discipline brings to the issue a different perspective, all of which should be taken into consideration when dealing with the thorny problems of ethics. Furthermore, this independence, which prevents any one player from seeing the whole picture, often leads to a lack of appropriate decision making, leaving the patient in the lurch.

The disadvantages of professional isolation, the problem with this model, are best illustrated by examining clinical situations that truly involve a multidisciplinary team in the care of one patient. Consider the difficulties encountered in attempting to make treatment decisions about an infant with Down's syndrome, complicated by severe cardiac abnormalities and duodenal atresia. The pediatric surgeon called in to consult on the case is concerned with and knows all the details of the child's surgical problem. The mother's primary nurse has learned that the parents are having severe marital problems, which have been exacerbated by the birth of this ill child, and she is trying to assist the parents to begin therapy. The obstetrician who cared for the mother during the antenatal period and delivered both this and a previous child is well acquainted with her history of severe postpartum depression and is monitoring her at present. Clearly, all players have important jobs to do in their special areas, but all of their information will be urgently needed and should be shared in order to make humane treatment decisions for the child.

The Health Squad Model

Most medical and allied health textbooks repeatedly refer to the "health team." While it is clear that the ideal way of contracting with other health professionals is to work *with* them in some way, there may be something just a little bit idealistic about this concept. Thus, we like to refer to this approach to interprofessional care as the "health squad model," a squad being defined as a group of persons organized for the performance of a specific function, in this case the provision of high quality health care. (However, because of its popularity, you will see references to the health team later in the book.) One of the basic requirements for the health squad approach to work is that each discipline must have genuine respect for the others (more about this in Chapter 15). If we accept this as our model, we are telling the patient that we aim to give the best of each discipline and that any ethical advice forthcoming will be based on appropriate input from a variety of people, each with something unique to offer. Another ideal perhaps, but essential as we head toward a century in which consumers will become even more concerned about and involved with their own health care.

Summary

When we enter into any occupational field, whether in law, accounting, business, nursing, medicine or any other, we accept certain cultural requirements of our chosen profession. While the delineation of responsibilities may often be job-specific, our representation of our profession and our contract with society is more general. Codes of professional ethics have been developed during the past one hundred years or so to define the responsibilities of these contracts and to guide appropriate behavior. Clearly, codes of ethics are not the only guidelines for ethical decision making, but they may be viewed as a first step. In addition to providing guidelines for our relationships with patients, these codes also help to define our relationships with other health professionals both inside and outside our own disciplines.

Questions for Discussion and/or Review

1. What advantages and disadvantages do codes of ethics offer to the individual health professional?

2. Is it possible for codes of ethics to reflect community opinion? Is it even necessary?

3. Which model of interprofessional care provides the best care for patients in your opinion? Why? Have you observed examples in the clinical area?

4. In which model would you prefer to work? Why?

5. Design and describe a model of health care delivery that you think would best assure humane and efficient patient care.

Recommended Reading

Kennedy, Ian. "Rethinking Medical Ethics," *Journal of the Royal College of Physicians and Surgeons of Edinburgh*, 27 (January, 1982), 1–8.

Levine, Myra. "Nursing Ethics and the Ethical Nurse," *American Journal of Nursing*, 77 (May, 1977), 845–847.

Veatch, Robert M. "Medical Ethics," *Journal of the American Medical Association*, 252 (October 26, 1984), 2296–2300.

3

That Unique Connection: A Relationship with a Patient

In this chapter:

■ The nature of the relationship between caregivers and patients

■ Pitfalls to avoid

■ Models of communication
- Parent/child
- Salesperson/customer
- The team

■ Hazards to the relationship

...the arrival of a new medical "style" and the turning inward of a whole generation of patients, have filled the consultation with anger and weakened the doctor's healing hand.

from *Bedside Manners: The Troubled History of Doctors and Patients* by Edward Shorter, 1985

When author Edward Shorter examined the disturbing changes in the doctor-patient relationship and described the historical roots of this "new" relationship, he was describing not only the individual patient's relationship to his/her personal physician, but also, in a broader sense, to the whole field of modern health care. In effect, the changes directly affecting the doctor/patient relationship that have been discussed in the literature and popular press can just as easily be applied to the relationship of the patient to any health care professional.

It is now common knowledge that more lawsuits are brought against doctors and hospitals as a result of breakdown in communication than because of clinical incompetence or negligence. Thus, it should be clear to you, the health professional, that our relationships with patients play a fundamental role in our ability to deal with any kind of problem requiring patient input—and today that involves almost everything. Clearly, dysfunctional relationships with patients can seriously complicate ethical dilemmas. If the patient is to be a serious partner in making health care decisions, the relationship between patient and caregiver must function well.

Many outside influences have conspired to change the way patients relate to their health care providers. Such developments as patients' rights, increased litigation, health care's high media profile and, to an enormous extent, high-technology medicine, which can place enormous obstacles (such as large machines!) between the health care worker and the patient, have affected that relationship which has, for centuries, been the cornerstone of health care. This is not to say that it has always been an easy relationship although, historically, the problems were different. A writer for *Time* magazine put it this way: "Never have doctors been able to do so much for their patients, and rarely have patients seemed so ungrateful" (Gibbs, 1989, p. 29).

The Nature of the Patient/Caregiver Relationship

Before we can examine in greater detail those factors that have changed our relationship with patients, we need to look first at the nature of this unique human connection. One way of examining the relationship is to look at the distance between us and our patients.

Measuring the Distance between Us: Professional Objectivity vs. Caring Compassion

The difference between a personal and a professional relationship is a question of distance and emotion. Of course, our relationships with patients must be professional, not personal, but what does that specifically mean?

A personal relationship is characterized by physical and emotional closeness and is a clearly inappropriate model for use with patients. The limited number and extent of the contacts between an individual health professional and a patient on a daily basis automatically precludes this personal closeness. Even if such closeness could be achieved, it would inevitably lead to burnout.

Some health care workers characterize the ideal professional relationship with a client as impersonal, distant, and coolly competent. This allows them to maintain objectivity in the face of often emotionally draining health care problems and ethical dilemmas, while protecting their own psyches from the potential trauma inherent in the healing relationship. There has to be something better, though, than cool competence. Patients expect more humanity in the delivery of their health care.

Ideally, your relationship with the patient should blend those qualities that are held in high esteem by health care professionals, such as knowledge, technical ability, efficiency, objectivity, and competence, with the human qualities of warmth, understanding, and compassion. It is essential to possess the ability to see the patient's side of an issue without taking on the problems as your own. The relationship should be that of one human being to another human being.

Professional Pitfalls

There are times, however, when it is advisable to distance yourself from the patient, while at the same time maintaining the therapeutic relationship. Some situations in which to be careful are described below.

- A patient is lonely. The health care worker who does not put some distance between him/herself and the lonely patient runs the risk of constant demands for companionship. It can be very tempting to the compassionate individual to try to do everything possible to help alleviate a person's loneliness, sometimes even at the risk of jeopardizing commitment to other patients. This temptation must be resisted.
- You feel pity for the patient. A pitiable patient is an emotional minefield for the health care worker. Pity resembles compassion, but it also can awaken grief or pain. This grief that you may feel for the pitiable patient endangers your objectivity and leads to personal trauma for you that will, again, ultimately affect others in your care.

- You overidentify with a patient. This problem arises when you have had a similar experience to that of the patient. You may believe that your past experience makes you better able to handle the situation; in fact, it is more likely to cloud your objectivity and lead you to impress your own values upon the patient as you attempt to do what is best, possibly, to solve your own, rather than the patient's, problem.
- The patient is a social acquaintance or a family member. It is almost impossible to be truly professionally objective in dealing with people who are well known to you and with whom you also have a personal relationship. The personal aspects of your relationship cannot be fully left outside the health care encounter and, while they may help certain aspects of the relationship, they will affect your ability to give objective advice. Thus, except in the case of an emergency, you should avoid these patients.

Professional distance is a concept that should never be confused with taking an impersonal approach to a patient. The human encounter between health care professional and patient is inescapably personal at its core. It is at this personal core where the health professional must begin to see the patient with all the respect that he/she would expect in the same circumstances.

Unequal Power

In spite of the fact that patients are better educated about health care than ever before and are increasingly more demanding, there is still an imbalance in the power structure of the relationship between patient and health care worker. By virtue of the fact that the health care system has something that the patient *needs* and that only the health care worker can provide access to what is needed, the patient is placed in a vulnerable position, dependent upon the health care worker. The patient is thus in an unequal position with the health care worker, a point that must be remembered and weighed very carefully in each encounter with a patient. As it is unlikely that this power imbalance will change, the health care worker needs to work with this and understand its dynamics.

The old adage that "knowledge is power" illuminates one of the major factors that creates this imbalance. The health care worker has knowledge and skills that the patient does not have and cannot easily acquire, and thus has a tool that can sometimes be used to effect compliance. Some modern patients may resent this expertise and many attempt to obviate it by demanding more information from the health professional. This sharing of information, while not equalizing the relationship, enables the patient to take more responsibility for his/her own health care.

In spite of the increased emphasis on patient autonomy in recent years, this power imbalance remains. Traditionally, both the medical and lay literature have discussed this imbalance as a component of the doctor/patient relationship but, with the ever-widening circle of health care providers, this power imbalance is now evident in the relationships between patients and virtually every other member of the so-called health team.

> It is doubtful that medical personnel would themselves like to be treated shabbily and impersonally. It is doubtful that they would like to be treated as though they were so unintelligent that it would be useless to offer them honest and helpful information. It is doubtful that they would like to be treated as voyeurs of their own care rather than participants in their healing experience. In short, it is doubtful that medical personnel would like to be treated the way many of them treat their patients. (Inlander, Levin, and Weiner, 1988, pp. 189–190)

In spite of the fact that some patients may still find comfort and security in assuming the dependent role when dealing with the health care system, there are many others who would echo the above sentiments expressed by the authors of the book, *Medicine on Trial*, a scathing view of contemporary medicine and its relationship with its patients. Health care workers would be well advised to acquaint themselves with these and similar views and to remember such accusations when examining their own practices. It is clear that an awareness of and sensitivity to this power imbalance is the first step in the health care worker's ability to respect the patient's autonomy.

Models of Communication in the Relationship

If the relationship with the patient is the cornerstone of health care delivery, then the keystone is communication. In its broadest sense, communication can really be only one-way or two-way. In one-way communication, the flow of information is in one direction only, with the individual in the power position usually providing the information. In contrast, the two-way communication model provides for a flow of information in both directions and relies on feedback from one source to the other and vice versa.

The following models delineate the possible configurations of communication in your relationship with the patient.

Parent/Child

In simpler times, this model described the traditional relationship with the patient, and it still exists today. The health care worker believes that he/she knows what is best for the patient, and the patient either believes it also or is too intimidated by the system to make any resistance known. While overt conflicts may occur less frequently under this model, the quality of the care provided may suffer, given the lack of patient input and autonomy. This relationship provides a clear example of paternalism in the health care system.

Salesperson/Customer

In this model, the objective of the relationship is that the customer (the patient) obtain the care that he/she thinks is needed and that he/she is demanding. The salesperson (the health care worker) sells what expertise he/she has to sell. Obviously, persuasive communication on the part of the salesperson is often required to make this surprisingly common model function, but it is usually quite easy to convince an intimidated customer that the knowledgeable salesperson is right. Unlike the parent/child interaction, the outcome of each encounter of this nature is dependent upon the abilities of both the salesperson *and* the customer to attain their goals. However, when their goals are divergent, this can be a very complicated relationship.

The Team

In this model, as in sports, all parties must agree on the goal of the encounter, in this case the necessary health care. There is an implied contract and a respect for one another's ability to make a contribution to the achievement of the common goal. Although the decision making is shared, the onus is on the health care worker(s) to provide the patient with needed information and then to listen to and act upon the patient's response. All parties must hold up their ends honestly. There are no stars here, only partners in care.

Obviously, this last situation describes an ideal relationship for dealing with ethical dilemmas. It is true, however, that not all patients are comfortable with the new responsibility this model entails and have difficulty dealing with the expectation that they will be partners in their care. It is the responsibility of the health care worker to ensure that the patient understands the expectations from the outset.

We have examined the micro-level concerns of your relationship with the patient, but what about the broader picture? What about the outside influences that we alluded to earlier? How important are they on a person-to-person level?

Hazards to the Relationship between Patient and Health Care Worker

As times have changed, the sanctity of the health care worker's relationship with the patient has changed as well—only too often it appears that this precious bond is being destroyed little by little. We present five modern phenomena that have had an enormous impact on that relationship and have contributed in no small measure to the ethical dilemmas facing us every day.

The Media

Many North Americans obtain most of their health information from the media. With reporters and other writers serving as middle men between the health care system and the patient, the opportunities for misinformation, misinterpretation, and general confusion are innumerable. Media coverage of medical research has resulted in health care consumers who are semiliterate regarding the new technologies, and what they lack in accurate, unbiased information, they make up for in enormous and often unfounded expectations as to what modern health care delivery can and should do for them. The North American patient who reads the newspaper even intermittently, scans a magazine once in a while, watches the evening news on television, or listens to the radio newscasts while driving to work every day is much more likely to learn about heart transplants than hemorrhoids. And yet, the number of people who can benefit from information about hemorrhoid treatment far outstrips the number of individuals who will legitimately present as heart transplant recipients. Transplantation, however, is far more glamorous than proctology.

Another aspect of the media's potential impact on our relationships with our patients is directly related to how members of our individual professions are depicted in the public arena. For example, doctors and/or nurses are frequently covered in the press as a consequence of either malpractice suits or strikes. It is hardly surprising, then, that patients' initial impressions of modern nurses and doctors may be less than pleasant and their reactions negative. Health care workers need to be aware of how they are painted in the press and how media images may color their relationships with patients, even creating hostility to be overcome.

Threat of Litigation

The alarming increase in the number of medical malpractice suits in recent years is taking its toll on the trust that must underlie our relationships with patients. As health care professionals, we are constantly aware that an unhappy patient, regardless of the cause of that unhappiness, more and more frequently considers litigation as the solution to the problem. This development makes health care workers wary and can erode the bond between us and our patients. Remember, as was previously mentioned, that more lawsuits are brought before the courts as a result of poor communication than for any other reason. This becomes important in making judgments when dilemmas are presented. Is avoidance of a possible lawsuit a factor that should be considered in making patient care decisions or giving advice? Consider the patient who presents at the office of the family doctor with a recurrent headache.

After a careful history and physical examination, it is clear to the doctor that the headaches are triggered by stressful events in the patient's life and can be quite easily relieved by comfort measures that the doctor has previously discussed with the patient. The patient, however, has just read a newspaper article about the local hospital's new CT scanner and the backlog of patients waiting for their examinations. The patient wants a CT scan. In the doctor's opinion, there is no medical indication for this diagnostic test. However, if the doctor fears litigation and has the slightest doubt about his/her diagnosis, there may be a tendency to acquiesce to the patient's demand to avoid possible future malpractice accusations. Surely this concern about litigation paints the picture for the doctor in a completely different color.

Patients' Rights Movement

As discussed in Chapter 1, the rise of consumerism in the marketplace in general is also having an impact in the health care industry. Acknowledgement of patients' rights has affected how health professionals relate to patients; their demands for accountability have changed how patients approach health care providers. Trust has frequently been replaced by skepticism, suspicion, and lack of faith. However, this growing consumer interest in health has positive results as well. In fact, this interest has often had the effect of making the patient much more willing to be accountable for his/her own decisions affecting his/her health. Health care workers can use this new awareness to the advantage of the relationship and the care provided. Patients' rights groups, for example, have spearheaded the move toward use of the living will.

Competition in the Health Care Marketplace

As more and more doctors graduate from medical school, more and varied allied health professionals find their niches, more nurses demand greater responsibility in the delivery of primary care, and more hospitals become more competitive, fear of losing patients becomes a very real concern for those professionals providing care to individual patients. There is no question that economic restraints in the health care system have resulted in the need to view patients, at least some of the time, in terms of the income that they represent. It is obvious that if this mind-set gets out of hand, another dimension will have entered into the relationship with the patient, one that has nothing to do with the best interests of the patient. In the end, patient care may be compromised.

However, from the patient's point of view, this competition to attract them could be advantageous. Health care workers have begun to realize that they must demonstrate more concern for the satisfaction of their patients by providing them with specialized services and listening carefully to what they have to say—a part of the communication process that has been frequently overlooked.

Modern Medical Technology

The final and perhaps most important of the developments eroding our relationships with patients is rapidly advancing technology. At the beginning of the twentieth century, the health care system was essentially unable to "cure" disease. However, as technology and pharmacology advanced, it became possible not only to alleviate suffering, but also to provide many patients with a cure. Obviously, this is a very welcome development, but it has interfered with the trusting relationship that formerly characterized the health care encounter.

The rapidly increasing knowledge base of medicine and health care has had a number of effects. First, health care professionals have had to scurry to keep up and continually ensure that their knowledge is truly current. This sometimes results in overinvestigation in an effort not to miss anything. Unnecessary tests may be administered, and/or patients may be subjected to unpleasant procedures when no clear need is demonstrated. The second effect of this advancing technology is that both patients and health care workers have begun to value highly what has come to be known as "quick-fix" medicine, for everything from a hangnail to heart disease. This reliance on high-tech medicine has moved the emphasis from the art of medicine to the science of medicine and has caused an impersonal wedge to come between patients and their caregivers.

As high-technology equipment physically distances the caregiver from the patient with a resulting lack of "hands-on" medicine, often the patient as a person seems to have been fragmented into body parts, chemicals, and electro-magnetic energy, to name but a few. With such a variety of health professionals delivering tests and treatments at each stage, it has become more and more difficult for any one individual to relate to the patient as a whole. No doubt this is one of the reasons for the increasing popularity of "holistic" health care.

There is a tale that has been told and retold of a biomedical engineer who was called into the intensive care unit by a physician to look at a cardiac monitor that was not working properly. Arriving promptly, the engineer began his examination at the electrical outlet, working slowly back toward the patient who was in the adjoining room. When he arrived at the bedside he found that the patient was dead. No one had noticed that the reason the machine was recording nothing was because there was nothing to record. While it sounds ludicrous that this could happen in a modern hospital, reliance on machines has distanced nurses, technicians, and doctors alike from the very people they have committed to care for. Similar scenes are played out every day, perhaps in less dramatic contexts.

Modern Hazards Threatening the Sanctity of the Relationship between Caregiver and Patient

- Pervasiveness of mass media

- Caregivers' fear of litigation

- Rise of consumerism

- Competition for patients

- Technological advances

Figure 3.1.

Summary

In every encounter with a patient there is a component which is medical or physiological in nature, but there is also a more important component that is neither. That element is the value systems that both you and your patient bring to the relationship, independent of one another. Further, your own understanding of relationships in general and communication in particular will affect the outcome of that encounter and determine how much the patient will trust you. A careful consideration of the modern wedges that threaten to widen the gap between caregiver and patient is necessary to the continued development of our abilities to deliver humane and compassionate care.

Questions for Discussion and/or Review

1. Describe your concept of the ideal relationship between caregiver and patient. What must be included? What must be avoided?

2. How could you incorporate your philosophy of patient care into your work?

3. What issues that may be important in making ethical decisions with a patient might you discuss during an initial interview?

4. Which model of communication do you prefer? As a caregiver? As a patient?

5. Discuss the advantages and disadvantages of each model of communication.

6. From your own experience describe health care situations which illustrate how each of the five obstacles discussed interfered with good relationships between caregivers and patients.

Recommended Reading

Benner, Patricia. *From Novice to Expert: Excellence and Power in Clinical Nursing Practice*. Menlo Park, California: Addison-Wesley, 1984.

Gibbs, Nancy. "Sick and Tired," *Time*, (July 31, 1989), 28–33.

Herzberg, Suzanne. "Client or Patient: Which Term is More Appropriate for Use in Occupational Therapy," *American Journal of Occupational Therapy*, 44 (June, 1990), 561–564.

Schafer, Arthur. "Dental Ethics: Getting the Balance Right," *Journal of the Canadian Dental Association*, 55 (March, 1989), 189–191.

Weston, W.W. "The Person: A Missing Dimension in Medical Care and Medical Education," *Canadian Family Physician*, 34 (August, 1988), 1701–1705, 1803.

4

Keeping Secrets: Confidentiality in Practice

In this chapter:

- ■ The nature and limits of confidentiality

- ■ Current factors which tend to erode confidentiality
  - Need for research data
  - Requirements of insurance companies and employers
  - Legal responsibilities of caregivers
  - Multidisciplinary health care system
  - Widespread use of computers
  - Public interest
- ■ The consequences of breaches in confidentiality

A sekret ceases tew be a sekret if it iz once confided—it iz like a dollar bill, once broken, it iz never a dollar again.

from *Affurisms,* Josh Billings, 1865

There is nothing more personal than confiding one's most intimate feelings, thoughts, fears, and anxieties to a member of the health professions. There are few things more tempting to a human being than to reveal or share a secret, and health professionals, for all their education and training, are only human. Neither doctors, nor nurses, nor any others who are entrusted with the most private secrets of other human beings are above yielding to this temptation from time to time. But, consider it from the patient's point of view. If you had the slightest reason to believe that your secrets were not safe with someone, you would think twice about mentioning them, even if withholding such information would be to the detriment of your care. There is no question that, as a component of the relationship with the patient, the concept of confidentiality deserves a chapter of its own.

Keeping information about the patient confidential has been expected of health care workers since the Hippocratic Oath. The International Code of Medical Ethics (1983) says that "a doctor owes to his patient absolute secrecy on all which has been confided in him or which he knows because of confidences entrusted to him." The International Council of Nurses Code (1973) says that "the nurse holds in confidence personal information and uses judgement in sharing this information." The American Medical Association's Principles of Medical Ethics (1980) says that the physician "shall safeguard patient confidences within the constraints of the law," and this last exhortation is echoed in many other modern codes.

Wait a minute! We started with a simple, clear, unequivocal statement to maintain confidentiality, evidently under any circumstances. What is all this waffling about using judgment and considering legal constraints? How much and what kind of judgment is to be exercised? To what extent are the laws of the land responsible for ensuring that we are ethical? Obviously, keeping patients' secrets is neither simple nor clear, and the codes that might guide our behavior are certainly open to interpretation.

The confusion about keeping patient confidences stems from those modern concerns that put the needs and rights of society at large before the needs of the individual patient. One current debate about the rights of AIDS patients to confidentiality, when weighed against society's right to know in order to avoid risk, provides us with a perfect example of the ethical dilemmas confronting us.

What Is Confidentiality?

Although the concept of confidentiality may seem simple to understand, there is more to it than meets the eye. For example, something that is confidential can be referred to as classified, restricted, undisclosed, secret, or private, and each of these terms has its own connotations. To understand the concept of confidentiality in the context of health care delivery, these questions require answers.

- What information is considered classified?
- To whom is access to this information restricted?
- Is a patient's secret still a secret when disclosed to another health professional?
- Does the patient always have a right to privacy?

Obviously, trust in their caregivers is essential if patients are to be relied upon to present all relevant information that might in any way affect their health care. Part of that trust is based on society's belief that the patient has the right to privacy, and everything that is disclosed to a health professional in the context of that relationship is a secret *unless it is necessary to disclose that information for the benefit of the patient or society.*

There is a great deal of controversy about this last consideration. We will discuss how that controversy developed and why the duty to *absolute* secrecy has required revision.

In 1948, the World Medical Association published what has come to be known as the *Declaration of Geneva.* It stated, quite clearly, "I will respect the secrets confided in me." At that time, there was no recognition of a physician's or any other health professional's duty to society. The dyadic nature of the relationship between the caregiver and the patient was absolute (Higgins, 1989).

Times have changed. Although the patient's right to privacy is still respected and the caregiver's obligation to maintain confidentiality is still expected, it is becoming more and more widely accepted that there are limits to an individual patient's right to privacy ("Medical Confidentiality," 1990). In other words, a reasonable claim to privacy cannot be made if concealment of information threatens others. An ethical dilemma arises when there is a disagreement about what information should be kept confidential and to what extent or to whom it should be revealed.

Factors Eroding Confidentiality

If we could follow a simple rule that told us never to break a patient's confidence, we would confront fewer ethical dilemmas. Unfortunately, such a dogmatic approach to ethics only paints us into a corner and removes a measure of our humanity. With this kind of approach, we would not break a patient's confidence even if other patients were in danger or if required to do so by law, as in the case of the elderly patient with deteriorating vision due to cataracts who refuses to give up driving a car. Rigid adherence to *never* breaking a patient's confidence under any circumstances would then provide an easy out, obviating the necessity to make a hard decision.

We now need to be aware of modern developments that have placed confidentiality in more jeopardy than ever before. We call these developments the "erosion factors" because of the nature of their effects on the exhortation to absolute secrecy in the caregiver/patient relationship. These developments cannot be ignored or forgotten, because they are not going to disappear.

Need for Research Data

Medical research is highly valued by society for its efforts to learn as much as possible about health and disease. In the pursuit of knowledge, however, information about real patients must be generated, and statistical information is often obtained retrospectively by examining hospital records. In fact, this is a daily occurrence in most large health care institutions. While health professionals are usually very conscientious about the requirement to avoid patient identifiers in the publication of this data, we must also consider the possibility that patients may wish that even those people engaged in extracting data from the charts not see their personal information. This need for medical data for purposes of research creates situations in which patient confidences might be broken.

Insurance Company Requirements

A second factor in the erosion of patient confidentiality is the need of the insurance industry to gain access to personal medical information about applicants for life and health insurance, and about accident victims. When applying for insurance, the individual patient gives the caregiver permission to provide the insurance company with the appropriate information. Occasionally, physicians, in particular, are tempted not to reveal certain facts to these companies in an ill-conceived attempt to save patients insurance dollars and in the belief that some information is strictly between doctor and patient. In spite of their good intentions, the practice is fraudulent and, if found out, can have detrimental consequences for the caregiver, the individual patient, and the future costs of insurance.

In the case of accident victims, insurance companies need to be certain that claims are not exaggerated. There have been instances in which companies have resorted to unauthorized means to obtain this confirmation. Caregivers who are asked for confidential patient information need to be sure that the patient has given authorization before providing such information.

Summary of Factors Contributing to the Erosion of Confidentiality

- Need for research data and statistics

- Insurance company requirements

- Occupational medicine requirements

- Third party interest

- Legal requirements

- Multidisciplinary nature of health care delivery

- Use of computers in health care

- Overriding public interest

Figure 4.1.

Occupational Medicine Requirements

Occupational medicine is also taking its bite out of patient confidentiality. In our increasingly complex world of work, employers often seem to think that they own their employees, body and soul. Physicians and other primary health care workers are more and more frequently confronted with the dilemma created by employers who insist on knowing minute details about a sick employee's health status. From the employers' point of view, they have a vested interest in the health of that individual as illness results in, at the very least, inconvenience, and frequently, increased costs to the business.

There is, however, a difference between dealing with an employer who is simply inconvenienced by an employee's illness and one who has a legitimate claim that certain illnesses might jeopardize the health or safety of others. It becomes a problem of ethics particularly where the law is unclear about the need to breach confidentiality. For example, in many areas of the offshore oil industry, individuals who are diagnosed as insulin-dependent diabetics are prohibited from working on oil rigs. Company policy states that it is the responsibility of the health professional conducting the pre-employment or periodic physical examination to report when the employee is unfit for work. Thus, to avoid a conflict between your values as a caregiver and the values of the company with which you are working, you need fully to be aware of and able to comply with the policies in an ethical manner.

Third Party Interest

Another hazard to patient confidentiality is third party involvement. Third party involvement refers to situations where an individual's rights may be breached by maintaining the confidentiality of another patient ("Medical Confidentiality," 1990). The most striking example of this dilemma today is found in the case of a patient who knows that he/she carries the AIDS antibody and refuses to tell those individuals in his/her life who might become infected without this knowledge. It is becoming increasingly obvious to most health professionals that the right of the third party to safety, especially in this case of risk of contracting a terminal disease, overrides the other party's right to privacy. The solution, however, is not so easy to put into practice. We discuss this further in a later chapter.

Legal Requirements

The concept of patient confidentiality is being further eroded by increasing legal requirements to break patient confidences. This is a difficult area that raises the question of whether something that is legal is ethical and vice versa. Ironically, the maintenance of confidentiality is not only an ethical obligation, but also a legal obligation. In spite of this, laws have more and more frequently created personal ethical dilemmas for health care professionals as they attempt to deal with the patients' right to privacy vs. the professionals' legal responsibilities to report.

One of the most commonly known laws involving an obligatory breach of patient confidentiality is that regarding the reporting of communicable diseases. These laws were enacted because of the belief that, in certain specified cases, the risk to society outweighed the individual patient's right to complete privacy. It may seem sensible for this information to be compiled and, if relevant, contacts to be followed up, yet the health professional needs to be aware that this breach of confidentiality may lead to consequences, such as the possible loss of individual liberty by forced confinement or forced treatment (Emson, 1988). This is not to suggest that these potential outcomes somehow negate the caregiver's responsibility to uphold the laws of the land, but all possible repercussions must be fully recognized.

There are other laws which require breach of absolute patient confidentiality. In some jurisdictions, the legal responsibility of the caregiver extends to reporting patient conditions that result in a hazard to other people. For example, in several US states and Canadian provinces, physicians are required by law to report to the department of motor vehicles the fact that an individual who holds a driver's licence has been diagnosed as epileptic. The consequence is that the individual patient's driver's licence will be revoked until the condition has been stabilized by medication for a certain period of time.

Suspected child abuse is another example of a situation in which a breach of patient confidentiality may be legally required. Recent laws in a number of jurisdictions require individuals with reason to suspect that a child is being abused to report this suspicion to the authorities. Although these laws usually extend beyond health professionals to cover anyone with this knowledge, clearly, health care professionals are in a key position to have access to physical evidence that might lead them to this belief.

Regardless of your opinion of how these legal requirements may encroach on personal liberties, as a health care provider, you need to consider not only your legal duty, but also the consequences to others.

Multidisciplinary Nature of Health Care Delivery

Another modern hazard to the patient's right to privacy is the increasing multidisciplinary nature of the health care system. Realistically, a patient entering a health care institution in North America today cannot expect that medical information about him/her will remain completely confidential.

> The old "rule" in the hospital was that "everyone has access to the patient's medical record except the patient"; the modern rule is that everyone (including the patient) has access. (Annas, 1989, p. 178)

The so-called team approach to delivery of health care is directly responsible for this particular breach of patient confidentiality. Quite apart from the inadvertent revelations that can be heard every day in the elevators and cafeterias of hospitals where health professionals unthinkingly discuss specifics of patient care for all to hear, the very fact that there are many specialized caregivers providing care means that increasingly large numbers of people have legitimate access to patient information. The more people who have access to the patient's medical record, the further afield the secrets will invariably travel.

Annas (1989) reports on a small survey carried out by a physician who decided to count the number of hospital personnel with legitimate access to an individual patient's chart. His total came to "at least 75 people"—6 attending physicians, 12 members of the house staff (interns and residents), 20 members of the nursing staff (this covered 3 shifts), 6 respiratory therapists, 3 nutritionists, 2 clinical pharmacologists, 4 unit secretaries or ward clerks, 15 students of various sorts, 4 hospital financial officers, and 4 chart reviewers (utilization, quality assurance, tissue review, and insurance auditor). While this number might seem inflated, particularly for some patients, an informal survey of the charts in areas where you work will indicate that large numbers of people do, indeed, have access to patient information. Today's patient needs to know that information must be given to other health team members for the care to progress as planned. The question an individual caregiver needs to answer for him/herself is: how much of what I know about a patient needs to be made known to others? Obviously, while the answer will vary from one situation to another, the question needs to be considered in each case.

Use of Computers in Health Care

Computers in health care are here to stay, and the potential threat to confidentiality they pose may be one of the most significant problems in their applications.

> It is possible where computerised medical records are involved to gain access to vast amounts of medical data at a stroke; moreover, this data could be of use in certain situations outside of medicine (for example, to the police or insurance companies). (deDombal, F.T., 1987, p. 183)

To what extent is this an important concern to individuals who operate computers in health care? Responsibility falls to those who hire computer specialists in health care to ensure that they understand that patient confidentiality is a fundamental part of health care delivery and must be maintained.

Overriding Public Interest

A recurring theme throughout this discussion has been the movement away from a strictly patient-centered confidentiality ethic toward concern for society at large. This need to consider the overriding public interest is perhaps the most perplexing of the issues that have eroded, and will continue to erode, patient confidentiality. Every day, the conflict between the public interest and the individual patient's interest seems more apparent. The psychiatrist or psychiatric nurse who believes that a disturbed patient is likely to harm others, or the counsellor who learns that a male prostitute who is HIV positive continues to ply his trade, or the family doctor who learns that a truck driver is a cocaine addict all have a serious dilemma in common. They have to balance the patient's right to confidentiality with the public's right to safety. Although there are still those who believe that the individual's rights always outweigh society's safety, this attitude is changing as we are faced with more and more of these situations. The absolute nature of confidentiality in the patient-caregiver relationship is no longer obvious.

General Effects of the Erosion Factors of Patient Confidentiality

When viewed as a whole, it may appear that our time-honored practice of keeping patient confidences hasn't much of a chance in modern health care. However, the detrimental effects of these erosion factors are so serious that we still must value highly the secrecy inherent in the traditional relationship with the patient.

First, the relationship of caregiver with patient has been profoundly altered. There are now so many factors that come between the caregiver and the patient that trust, the cornerstone of the encounter, may give way to skepticism or distrust on the part of the patient. Second, as a result of distrust, patient care may suffer. A patient who believes that his/her secrets are not safe with a caregiver is likely to withhold information that might be essential to the diagnosis and treatment of a particular condition. Most patients are not in a position to make judgments about what is and what is not relevant and thus cannot be left to make those kinds of decisions. Clearly, patients need to know what you, as the caregiver, believe in and do about confidentiality in practice.

However, the patient has a right to know that there are limits to the extent of the confidentiality of the encounter. In situations like some of those described above, this needs to be made very clear. On the other hand, some patients have given little thought to the fact that you will maintain their confidences and fail to realize that you will need special authorization to break that confidence. Failing to tell patients this can sometimes result in a breakdown in communication, especially in situations where failure to disclose information to an employer has had unpleasant effects for the employee.

Summary

Human values change over time and throughout the society from which they emerge. Respect for the concept of patient confidentiality is no different from placing a high value on honesty or telling the truth, and the extent to which any of these can be put into practice is dependent upon the times. Times have changed and so too has the value placed on the patient-centered ethic. Our concerns today are broader than they once were, and our solutions to these dilemmas need to strike a balance between two positions—absolute secrecy and the greater good of society.

Questions for Discussion and/or Review

1. Under what circumstances and for what reasons do you think that patient confidentiality must be broken? Give several specific examples.

2. As a health care consumer (which we all are) how do you feel about the need to consider the safety of society rather than the individual's right to privacy under certain circumstances?

3. Is it ever permissable for health professionals to comment about colleagues or patients to other patients or visitors? Under what circumstances?

4. What negative results do you think might flow from a breach of confidentiality? How would you deal with an irate patient over this issue?

5. Does the right of patients (or, in some cases, their families) to see their charts affect the way you record information?

Recommended Reading

Annas, George J. "Privacy and Confidentiality," in *The Rights of Patients: The Basic ACLU Guide to Patient Rights*, 2nd ed., Carbondale and Edwardsville: Southern Illinois University Press, 1989, pp. 175–195.

Emson, H.E. "Confidentiality: A Modified Value," *Journal of Medical Ethics*, 14 (June, 1988), 87–90.

Higgins, Gerald L. "The History of Confidentiality in Medicine: The Physician-Patient Relationship," *Canadian Family Physician*, 35 (April, 1989), 921–926.

5

Informed Decision Making

In this chapter:

- ■ The nature of informed consent

- ■ Who should obtain consent

- ■ When consent is necessary

- ■ Prerequisites of informed consent
  - Mental competence
  - Adequate information
  - Voluntary choice
- ■ Special problems
  - Emergencies
  - Inadequate grasp of information

Volenti non fit iniuria [To a person who consents, no injustice is done].

Legal maxim

The Nature of Informed Consent

Consent is a concept that has been defined in many different ways. For example, the term has been used to mean voluntary agreement, voluntary yielding, acquiescence, and even compliance, implying one individual giving in to the will of another. In the context of modern health care, informed consent is the essential element of patient autonomy and, unfortunately, creates a whole host of ethical dilemmas. It is one of the most misunderstood concepts in modern health care ethics, on the part of both the caregiver and the patient.

Ethics and the law are two different things, but are, indeed, closely related. Probably nowhere else in biomedical ethics are these two more closely intertwined than in the issue of informed consent. To help understand the concept and how it works in practice, let's go back to Dr. Moral for a minute.

If you will recall, Dr. Moral is a busy family physician who seems to encounter his fair share of ethical dilemmas, whether he recognizes them or not. Today, he must follow up on one of the encounters he had when we first met him. Despite the fact that he, himself, has reservations about the necessity of routine circumcision of newborn baby boys, he has agreed to do the procedure for one of his partners who refuses to do them and has little experience in doing them anyway. According to what Dr. Moral reads in the chart, it is the wish of the patient that her son be circumcised because her husband is circumcised. Dr. Moral finishes reading Mrs. White's chart, picks up a routine hospital consent form, fills in the blanks regarding the procedure, and heads for her room.

"Mrs. White, I'm Dr. Moral. Dr. Fence has asked me if I might do your son's circumcision. I'd like to talk to you about it first."

"Are you going to try to talk me out of it too?"

"What I would like to do is explain the risks to you so that you can make an informed decision about whether or not you want it done," he replies.

"I already told Dr. Fence that I want my son circumcised. My husband is circumcised and he wants our son done as well. So let's dispense with the medical double-talk and get on with it."

Dr. Moral wonders how Dr. Fence had approached the situation and is concerned that Mrs. White isn't going to listen to what he has to say, but he proceeds with his explanation anyway. She signs the consent form and he goes away to make the arrangements, all the while wondering if she is really the one who wants this procedure done at all and if she has, indeed, made an informed decision.

As he reaches for the telephone in the nursing station on the postpartum floor to call the nursery, he overhears a resident and a nurse in conversation.

"Susan, take this down and get Mrs. Johnson to sign for her arteriogram, will you? You know all about these things."

The nurse takes the consent form handed to her and says, "Are you sure you shouldn't be getting this yourself?"

"Listen, I thought you nurses with your university degrees could explain all these things to patients without our help."

"Okay, okay," she says. "I can probably do a better job than you can anyway." She takes the consent form and leaves the desk.

As Dr. Moral waits on the telephone on hold, it occurs to him that the nurse is probably right. She probably does know more about patient teaching than the resident does and probably has a higher opinion of the value of that teaching, but she is not the one who will be doing the procedure. Oh well, he thinks, that's the way things are done.

Again, in the course of a normal day, Dr. Moral has just faced several ethical problems which involve not only patients, but also other health care personnel, and all of which revolve around the issue of informed consent.

It is important for all caregivers to ask themselves the following questions.

- What does it really mean for the patient to give "informed consent"?
- Which health professional should be obtaining consent?
- How does one really obtain that consent?
- When a patient's wishes conflict with what, in the opinion of the caregiver, is in his/her best interests, how can free consent be obtained?

Is There Such a Thing as Informed Consent?

The idea that an adult human being should have some say in the decisions that will affect his/her body is rooted in legal precedents in the United States of the early 1900s. However, the actual phrase, *informed consent,* was coined in the California Court of Appeal in 1957 (Silverman, 1989). The case in question involved a patient who had suffered permanent paralysis following a surgical procedure and who claimed that the physicians were negligent and that they had failed to inform him of the risk of paralysis. In the judgment, the judge referred to a new duty of disclosure, tempered with discretion, and coined the phrase "informed consent," which has stuck ever since.

The Purpose of Informed Consent

The term, "informed consent," however, is misleading. The purpose of providing information to patients is to give them the necessary basis of knowledge so that they can make decisions about their health care, *not so that they may be persuaded to do what the caregiver thinks is best for them.* Actually, a more useful term to use might be "informed decision making," which describes more accurately the process that an autonomous patient, who has been given all reasonable information, goes through in making his/her own decisions. This patient, in fact, may even refuse the proffered procedure rather than consent to it.

Who Should Obtain Consent for What?

This question may seem fairly straightforward to you: the person who will perform the procedure ought to inform the patient of what he/she needs and wants to know and should obtain the patient's written consent. However, in this day of multidisciplinary health care and levels of care within each discipline, the answer is not so clear.

In one of the situations presented at the beginning of the chapter, Dr. Moral overheard a typical conversation in a teaching hospital in which a doctor asked a nurse to get a patient's signature for an arteriogram. Many a nurse has been asked to obtain a patient's written consent for diagnostic procedures or treatment that she/he will not personally carry out. The same is true of other allied health workers, such as respiratory therapists and physiotherapists, among others. Sometimes, the nurse is also expected to explain the procedure to the patient, but most hospital consent forms stipulate that the procedure has been explained *by the physician who will do the procedure.* If asked by a doctor to obtain consent, should the nurse comply with the doctor's request?

In view of the legal ramifications, it is probably in neither the nurse's nor the doctor's best interests if the nurse complies. From an ethical standpoint, the nurse needs to be convinced of the informed nature of the consent. To uphold the patient's right to self-determination, the nurse needs to know that the patient has received enough understandable information on which to base an informed decision. If the procedure is medical in nature and is to be performed by a physician rather than a nurse or therapist, then, although the other health professionals may be able to explain further to the patient, the doctor should be the one who gives the basic information and actually sees the decision carried through.

Difficulties arise in situations where there are several layers of doctors dealing with individual patients. For example, in teaching hospitals, final-year medical students, interns, residents at any stage of their education, and staff doctors, as well as additional consultants, are frequently involved in any one case. Thus, a number of medical personnel, not to mention other health professionals, may all be involved in a procedure for which patient consent is required by law. The person in charge bears the ultimate responsibility for conveying information, but from an ethical point of view, in order to allow the patient to make a fully informed choice, each person involved has a responsibility to ensure that this has, indeed, been done.

The question of what needs to be consented to is another issue. Each procedure, whether diagnostic or therapeutic, that is carried out for the patient's health needs to be *chosen* by the patient after appropriate instruction. Each hospital has its own policies regarding inclusive consents which may be obtained by a clerk in the admitting office. In the past, these consents have given blanket permission for routine tests, such as blood taking, in order to avoid assault and battery charges; patients were rarely asked to consent to individual blood tests. This, however, has changed since the appearance of AIDS. As a consequence of the nature of the reactions to positive AIDS antibody tests, hospital policies usually dictate that individual consents be obtained for this test. Patient autonomy is respected as the patient, knowing the consequences of his/her action, makes an informed choice. The ethical dilemma that this presents, however, is that allowing the patient to make this informed choice robs the caregiver of the choice to determine whether or not the needs and rights of society at large overrule the individual patient's right. This is a very dramatic example of how the traditional patient-centered ethic poses significant problems in today's complicated health care world.

The Prerequisites to Informed Consent

Three elements must be in place if the patient is to make an informed choice.

- The patient must have the mental capacity to make that choice.
- The patient must be properly informed.
- The decision must be voluntary.

Patient Competence

An individual is considered to be competent to give consent if he/she is able to understand the nature of the proposed treatment or procedure, its anticipated effects, its risks, and the alternatives to the proposed course, if any. However, a number of situations serve to complicate this relatively straightforward statement.

How old must a person be in order to be competent to consent? Traditionally, the age of majority under the law was considered to be the competent age; however, more and more frequently the courts are acting to uphold the right of individuals younger than this age to give their own consent, based on the belief that they are often able fully to comprehend the nature and effects of proposed beneficial treatment.

The next question that needs to be answered is what to do about an individual who has been judged to suffer from a mental incapacity. Legally, only the court can decide when someone else may consent to treatment on behalf of another adult, and this will only be granted in situations where there is clearly a benefit to the patient. For example, the court generally will not allow a third party to consent to a contraceptive sterilization on behalf of a mentally incapacitated adult as this procedure is usually not considered medically necessary. Its social utility, and perhaps its ethical rightness, may be quite a different matter.

In these cases, in the context of the actual decision itself, the ethical concerns about informed decision making are the same as if the individual were giving consent for his/her own treatment. The main difference, however, is that the decision is not based on what the proxy wants, but on what he/she believes the patient would want. The caregiver charged with asking for such consent should then word the question in such a way that the patient's wishes are given priority. For example, do not ask what the proxy would like you to do, but what the patient would want.

Adequate Information

In order for any patient to make a health care decision, it is essential that he/she be properly informed by the health professional(s). Both the information and the way in which it is given must be adequate. This requires high quality communication skills on the part of health professionals—something by no means guaranteed by training and licensure. If you recall, a lack of communication skills is responsible for most lawsuits against health professionals. Thus, the concept of informed decision making on the part of the patient is dependent upon our skills and relationships with patients.

This gives rise to the question of how much information is enough to convey to patients. Today, the standard against which this is measured, at least from a legal point of view, is by exercising judgment and what has come to be called the "reasonable patient" standard. The question to be answered is: what would a reasonable patient want to know given the same situation and circumstances (Gilmore, 1985). The individual caregiver must have the ability to make such a judgment. A caregiver should remember that what a reasonable patient would want to know may exceed, or at least be different from what, in a paternalistic health care system, was considered to be what the patient ought to know. In order to meet this requirement, in language that the patient understands, the caregiver must give the patient:

- a description of the proposed treatment;
- a description of its risks and benefits;
- an estimation of the probability of success;
- a description of the recuperation required;
- a description of the alternatives;

- an assessment of the probable results of no treatment;
- any other information other health professionals would provide to patients in similar situations (Annas, 1989).

Voluntary Consent

The requirement that the consent must be voluntary is a difficult one. How much and what kind of information, as well as how it is presented, can all affect the freedom with which the consent is given. For example, when a transplant coordinator obtains consent for organ donation from a bereaved family, is consent freely given without coercion if the family is told that a specific patient will die should they refuse? In this situation, the guilt generated in the family could be construed to be a form of coercion, thus failing to afford the family members the opportunity to exercise their autonomy. In addition, the caregiver's own values might be revealed in the choice of words used to present the alternatives to the patient and thus exert subtle pressure.

Special Problem Areas

There are always special situations where consideration must be given to modifying the practice of allowing the patient to make an informed decision.

Emergencies

In an emergency situation, where immediate action is necessary to save the patient's life, the decision to treat and how to treat is left up to the caregiver. Efforts to inform the patient in an attempt to allow the individual to make an informed decision about treatment options is academic if the patient dies.

Inadequate Grasp of Information

One of the major problems in our communication with patients is their frequent inability to recall the information given to them by a health professional (Cresswell, 1983). This is, of course, especially problematic in attempts to do the right thing by promoting informed decision making by patients. Many research studies have been carried out to determine patient recall of information presented to them by health professionals, and results have been very discouraging. One good example is a study of 20 chronic heart disease patients who, by all accounts, were generally better informed about their conditions than many other patients, because of the chronic nature of their illnesses. The patients all underwent heart surgery and were tested four to six months after the procedure to determine what, if anything, they could recall about the information they were given at the time that they signed consent for the surgery. None of them had a precise recollection of the content of the discussion, and two patients, who were tested ten days and six weeks after their surgery, could not even remember that the interview had taken place at all (Robinson and Merav, 1976).

Summary

Obviously, we need to take into account not only the legal conditions under which informed consent is to be obtained, but also more practical considerations that ensure ethical conduct in upholding patient autonomy. Patients today generally want to be informed about their conditions, but not all want to have an equal role in the decision making, and not all participate in the process equally well. Some researchers have indicated that the most important factor motivating people to give their consent to medical treatment is not their comprehension of the information presented to them in the consent procedure, but their confidence and trust in the physician and nurse (Bergler et al., 1980). Thus, skill in patient education is the most important factor in doing the right thing in this case.

Although encouraging informed decision making is part of our legal responsibilities, simply fulfilling the letter of the law is not enough. Properly informing patients is also one of our ethical responsibilities in order that we may help uphold the patient's right to autonomy in health care.

Questions for Discussion and/or Review

1. Why does the phrase "informed decision making" better describe the ideal process than "informed consent"?

2. When many health professionals are involved in a patient's case, who should obtain consent? Why?

3. For what procedures does your institution require consent? How do they specify it must be obtained?

Recommended Reading

Cahn, C.H. "Consent in Psychiatry: The Position of the Canadian Psychiatric Association," *Canadian Journal of Psychiatry*, 25 (February, 1980), 78–85.

Miller, Leslie J. "Informed Consent: I and II," *Journal of the American Medical Association*, 244 (November 7 and 21, 1980), 2100–2103, 2347–2350.

Schwartz, Robert and Andrew Grubb. "Why Britain Can't Afford Informed Consent," *Hastings Center Report*, (August, 1985), 19–25.

6

Patients' Rights and Responsibilities

In this chapter:

- ■ Characteristics of "rights"

- ■ Legal and moral rights

- ■ Patients' rights—what they are and what they are not

- ■ When conflicts arise

- ■ Patients' responsibilities
  - Disclosure
  - Compliance with medical regime
  - Maintenance of health

The Members of the Medical Profession, upon whom so many arduous duties are imposed, and who are required to make so many sacrifices of ease, comfort and health for the welfare of mankind, have certainly the right to expect that patients should entertain a just sense of duties which they owe to their medical attendants.

Code of Medical Ethics, as presented at the first annual meeting of the Canadian Medical Association,
September, 1868

Human rights, minority rights, women's rights, rights of the unborn, the right to life, the right to death and on and on—the litany of rights about which much has been written in both the lay and the professional literature seems to lengthen with each passing day. One of the more recent additions to this list is patients' rights. And the acceptance of this concept poses some of the most perplexing ethical dilemmas in health care—situations in which competing rights come into conflict. When faced with the reality of being unable to uphold everyone's rights, hard decisions have to be made.

There is however, another side to the rights issue. This is a side that has received much less attention than society's obligation or responsibility to grant and uphold these rights, and that is the obligations or responsibilities of the individual who holds those rights. Thus, it is our contention that, not only does the grantor of the right have an obligation, but so too does the holder of that right. This concept of reciprocal responsibilities has some very important implications for the practice of health care, and the caregiver's ability to make sound ethical decisions in practice depends on understanding it.

The Nature of Rights: Defining Patients' Rights

In Chapter 1 we discussed some current social trends that continue to have an impact on health care ethics. One of those trends is the rise of the consumer movement, which has had a direct effect on patient rights.

The push to have the concept of consumers' rights embedded in the provision of goods and services, including health care delivery, has formed the basis for the rather diffuse patients' rights movement in North America. According to the American Civil Liberties Union Handbook (Annas, 1989), "By demanding that patients be treated as unique human beings, the recognition of human rights in health care can humanize both the hospital and the encounters with physicians and other health care professionals" (p. xiii). Understanding and respecting the rights of the patient, then, can assist us, as health professionals, to put the art of caring back into the science of health care delivery.

Before we can exercise that respect, though, we need to understand what rights are in general, and what rights should be accorded to patients in particular. Rights are claims that individuals and groups can make upon others and upon society, but they are not merely claims—they are *justified claims.*

> A claim of a right invokes entitlements; and when we speak of entitlements, we mean not those things which it would be nice for people to have, or which they would prefer to have, but which they must have, and which if they do not have they may demand. (Fried, 1977, p. 68)

There is an important difference between legal and moral rights. Legal rights are those claims that are justified by the existence of current legal principles or rules. An individual who believes that his/her legal rights have been violated has recourse to the courts to determine if his/her judgment is accurate and, in addition, what retribution might be made.

In ethics, however, no matter how close the association to the law in a specific case, we are still dealing not with legal rights, but with moral rights. A moral right is a claim that is justified by current moral principles and rules. Therein lies the problem in health care delivery. A lack of consensus about morality in North American society underlies many disagreements about what rights patients have beyond those dictated by the law. In an attempt to understand further what rights are and how they are exercised, we need to examine the conditions under which they are exercised.

First, a right is not something that the holder of that right *must* exercise, but something that he/she may *choose* to exercise or not. If an individual has a right to a particular medical procedure to alleviate a medical problem, this means that the patient has the choice to accept the procedure or not.

Second, because we, as a society, or we, as health care professionals, have accorded specific rights to patients, we have the obligation to uphold those rights and to do everything that we can to make sure that the patient can exercise those rights. If, for example, we agree with some of the patients' rights associations and grant the patient the right to death with dignity, our institutional policies and our individual practices must reflect that right and be designed in such a way as to enable patients to achieve it.

Finally, a right must be available and enforceable. It would be ludicrous in health care delivery to suggest that patients have a right to services and treatment that are not available or, if available, that we cannot ensure that the patient will receive. If, for example, we suggest that each patient with end-stage heart disease who meets the medical criteria has the right to a heart transplant, we are being irresponsible because we cannot fully uphold that right. This treatment is too specific to be defined as a right. There are too many other variables over which we have no control that play a part in determining whether or not the patient will actually be able to receive that heart transplant. The best we can do is to grant the patient the right to equal consideration.

The misunderstanding of this condition by both patients and health professionals leads to enormous problems in health care ethics. Technological advances in medical care, coupled with increased consumer demand, have resulted in the belief that patients have rights of equal access to care, and this equal access has been defined in a very narrow and literal way. We need to broaden our understanding of this supposed right so that we can realistically carry out our obligations.

Some authors (Bandman and Bandman, 1990) have also suggested that another condition of a right is that if it is violated or overridden in some way, the patient should be given compensation. The problem with this suggestion is that, in practice, it is so difficult to exercise as to be worthless. For example, if a patient has a reportable sexually transmitted disease, his/her right to privacy must be overridden for the benefit of past or potential contacts, but there is little that can be done to compensate that individual for failing to completely uphold his/her right to privacy. And this situation clearly exemplifies the central problem with patients' rights. What do we do when one person's rights are in conflict with those of another person or with the rights of society?

What Rights Are We Talking About?

As health professionals we have a responsibility to know what rights patients possess in the context of the health care delivery system. We must consider these rights not only from our point of view, but also from the point of view of the patient. What rights can the health system grant? What rights do patients believe they have?

That patients' opinions of what their rights are might differ from that of health professionals may seem strange, but evidently that is exactly what is happening. If this were not so, and if society had the wherewithal to grant all rights that patients perceive they are entitled to, there would not have been such a proliferation of patients' rights groups throughout the US and Canada over the past two decades. It is extremely important for health professionals to be aware of these groups and to respect what they stand for.

For example, the National Health Federation, with its head office in California, is one of the oldest of the patients' rights organizations in North America. Founded in 1955, the association's mandate is to advocate "the absolute right of the people to enjoy the civil liberty of freedom of choice in matters of personal health where such choices do not infringe upon the liberties of others" (NHF Silver Anniversary

Summary of Conditions under which Patients' Rights are Exercised

- The exercise of any right is optional.

- The grantors of a right must allow the holders of the right to exercise it.

- A right must be accessible and enforceable.

Figure 6.1.

Booklet, 1970). It calls itself "a non-profit, consumer-oriented organization devoted exclusively to health matters."

The People's Medical Society is another high-profile patients' rights organization based in Allentown, Pennsylvania. According to their promotional literature, their philosophy encompasses the following:

- to give people the information they need to protect themselves in their daily lives; and
- to bring thousands of people together as a social and political force strong enough to stand up to the medical establishment.

Their strong words are backed by a board of directors that is impressive, even to the most narrow-minded health professional, and includes a chairman who is a professor at the Yale University School of Medicine and the director-general of the Health Promotion Directorate of Health and Welfare Canada. In addition, their book, *Medicine on Trial: The Appalling Story of Ineptitude, Malfeasance, Neglect and Arrogance* (Inlander, Levin, and Weiner, 1988), has received considerable public attention.

Other such groups have sprung up across the continent. Some of the objectives of these consumer-based groups are: to act as a patient advocate by assisting patients to get their grievances heard; to advocate easier and more equitable complaint procedures; and to promote public awareness of patients' rights within the health care system.

Here is a summary of what these groups believe to be some of the rights that patients can claim, including the right to:

- be treated with respect and have one's next of kin treated with respect;
- receive a reasonable response to requests for services;
- receive humane and efficient medical care;

- receive reasonable continuity of care;
- be informed of a health professional's personal morality if this may affect treatment;
- adequate information about one's disease;
- choose one's own medical therapy;
- not be subjected to unnecessary diagnostic procedures;
- not be emotionally exploited;
- privacy;
- a second opinion;
- death with dignity.

Patients are thinking seriously about their moral rights, and you need to be aware of and ready to consider what they may demand.

Whose Rights Take Precedence?

The belief that patients have rights seems to be self-explanatory. After all, western society is committed to upholding human rights. Both the US and Canadian constitutions provide protection under the law for human rights. Thus, since patients are human beings, logic tells us that they, too, have rights. In practice, the problems with the logic are two-fold.

First, as we have already discussed, the rights to which we refer in health care are often not legal rights, but moral rights, and the conditions under which they are exercised are not well understood by the patients. There are few moral laws that are universally accepted and that, if not followed, will result in retribution.

The second, and perhaps even larger problem in practice, is the fact that conflicts of rights happen every day. In such conflicts the rights of some people will take precedence over those of others, who will then be unable to exercise their rights. We must make the tough decisions about which rights will take precedence. We have already illustrated that an individual patient's right may conflict with that of another individual patient or with that of society. In equally perplexing situations, the right of the patient may conflict with a right of the health professional, such as an AIDS patient's right to be treated vs. a nurse's right to refuse care. So, how can decisions in these matters be made?

Much has been written about what criteria need to be considered when deciding which right takes precedence, but none of the methods is without problems in clinical practice. Figure 6.2 presents some of the questions whose answers will help in decision making.

We need to keep in mind, however, that even when the answers to these questions seem clear, controversies can still arise. One of the problems is the necessity,

Questions to Ask When Making Decisions about Conflicting Rights

- Are both claims really rights?

- How do you rate the relative importance of each claim?

- How do you rate the outcome of the exercise of each claim?

- Are the outcomes of the exercise of each right real or potential?

- How would you compare the motivation behind each claim?

- Which claim has a more positive social benefit?

- How would you compare the outcome of non-exercise of each claim?

Figure 6.2.

especially in rights conflicts, to see the problem more from a macro than a micro point of view—to see the bigger picture, in other words. For example, it may be easy for you to sit back in your office and say that, because resources are scarce, patients over the age of 70 are not entitled to access to renal dialysis. If, however, your 71-year-old father, who is otherwise quite spry, experiences kidney failure, you may suddenly decide that each situation needs to be considered on a case-by-case basis. Your lack of objectivity in this situation has resulted in your inability to see the bigger picture. In any event, it will always be hard to make decisions that deny care or treatment to some, and pressure from those excluded may be intense.

Patients' Responsibilities

It should be clear by now that in order for patients to exercise their rights, health professionals must assist them. While much has been written about how to do this, far less has been written about patients' responsibilities. In the past, however, more consideration was given to this area. The physicians who wrote the original draft of the Canadian Medical Association's Code of Ethics, quoted at the beginning of this chapter, obviously considered the idea important enough to rate special consideration in their code and defined some of the constituents of a "just sense of duties," some of which are still relevant today.

Disclosure of Information

First, patients have a responsibility to disclose all relevant information regarding their health status; they should be told that you expect them to fulfil this obligation if they expect you to provide optimum care. The trust that develops in the relationship between patient and caregiver and the understanding of the confidential nature of the interaction play a vital role in a patient's willingness to disclose information to health professionals.

Compliance with Medical Regime

If patients are to expect optimum health care as a right, they have a duty to comply with the medical regime, and you have a reasonable right to expect that compliance. This, however, is not quite the same as the precept found in the Canadian Medical Association's 1868 code of ethics when it counseled the patient that "obedience to the prescriptions of his [sic] physician should be prompt and implicit. He should never permit his own opinions as to their fitness to influence his attention to them" (C.M.A., 1868, article 2, section 6). Once a patient has agreed to be cared for by a particular caregiver and thus has entered into a type of contract, and after being given adequate information to make an informed choice, he/she has an obligation to follow through so that the caregiver can provide optimum care. Sometimes we need to make sure that patients are aware of this duty.

Maintenance of Health

Finally, it seems reasonable that if we believe everyone has a right to health care, each one of us should have some responsibility to keep as healthy as possible. Today, this means that patients have an obligation to take an active part in the maintenance of their health and that we can reasonably expect them to do this to the extent that they are able. Moreover, patients have a responsibility to be realistic about what health care can deliver to them. We, in the health professions, are guilty of creating often unrealistic expectations in health care delivery and need to be aware of this to avoid contributing further to it. Not everyone can or should have access to all that modern medical technology has to offer. Most caregivers would agree that, at the present time, in vitro fertilization (IVF) is a scarce resource that cannot be provided to every woman. Is the 42-year-old mother of three who underwent successful tubal ligation five years ago, has changed her mind about the completion of her family, and is now demanding IVF being realistic about what the health care system can and should provide to her? You decide.

Summary of Reasonable Patient Responsibilities

After patients have entered into the therapeutic relationship with a caregiver, they have a duty to:

- disclose all relevant information regarding their health status;

- comply with the medical regime;

- keep as healthy as possible.

Figure 6.3.

The concept of patient responsibilities under discussion—that health care consumers do, indeed, have a duty to keep in good health, must take responsibility for their actions, and should reasonably expect that if they fail to fulfil this obligation, their right to health care ought to be reduced accordingly—raises many problems. While encouraging the acceptance of these responsibilities may be an ideal toward which we strive, in practice it is difficult to act on the basis of these expectations. For example, when hospital beds are at a premium, should the individual who has smoked two packages of cigarettes a day, in spite of warnings from a health professional, have the same access to a bed as the person who has tried to fulfil his/her duty to keep healthy and who has succumbed despite all efforts? The obvious difficulty is in assigning values to health promotion and disease prevention practices.

Summary

Modern North Americans believe strongly in fundamental human rights, a concept that is embedded in the constitutions of both the United States and Canada. It seems reasonable, then, that the modern consumer of health care would expect to have certain rights within the health care delivery system. Caregivers need a solid understanding of what constitutes a right, how it is granted, and how it might be fulfilled in order to provide adequate care to all patients. On the other hand, it is also reasonable to expect that patients will fulfil their responsibilities, as well as exercise their rights.

Problems arise when acknowledged rights conflict with one another. So-called self-inflicted illnesses and non-compliance are situations where the rights of one individual interfere with the rights of others. While we may think that in practice we should leave these philosophical arguments aside and treat everyone in the same way, the crunch comes when resources are scarce. How do we make the hard decisions in allocating those resources? Then the theoretical scenario with its puzzling questions becomes all too real, as we shall see in the next chapter.

Questions for Discussion and/or Review

1. What are some important patient rights? Responsibilities?

2. Do you think the patients' rights movement has or has not been beneficial to the health care delivery system? Why or why not?

3. If and when you are a patient yourself, what rights would you exercise? What rights, if any, and under what circumstances, would you be prepared to give up?

4. Does the patient who abuses his/her own health (e.g. smoking, alcohol, or drug abuse) have the right to expect equal access to health care? Why or why not?

Recommended Reading

Brett, Allan S. and Laurence B. McCullough. "When Patients Request Specific Interventions: Defining the Limits of the Physician's Obligation," *New England Journal of Medicine*, 315 (November 20, 1986), 1347–1351.

Burgess, Michael M. "Ethical and Economic Aspects of Noncompliance and Overtreatment," *Canadian Medical Association Journal*, 141 (October 15, 1989), 777–779.

Coy, Janet. "Autonomy-Based Informed Consent: Ethical Implications for Patient Non-Compliance," *Physical Therapy*, 69 (October, 1989), 826–833.

7

Resource Allocation

In this chapter:

- ■ Causes of diminishing resources
  - Overuse
  - Patient demand
  - Media reports
- ■ Problems of resource allocation

- ■ Possible bases of resource allocation
  - Ability to pay
  - Past contribution to society
  - Potential contribution to society
  - Waiting in line
  - Individual need
- ■ The Oregon Solution

Let justice be done though heaven should fall.

                                                                        Proverb

It should be apparent by now that few ethical dilemmas in health care involve a direct choice between good and evil. If this were the case, practical ethics would be a simple matter. Much more common are situations involving hard choices between the lesser of two evils or between two conflicting goods. When two patients need to be admitted to intensive care, and both could benefit from that care, but there is only one bed available, which patient should be admitted? How is the decision to be made? This is the dilemma of resource allocation in health care delivery.

> The spectacular medical achievements of the past few decades have not only extended human life but have greatly enhanced the quality of that life. But the new, ultrasophisticated techniques that have prolonged so many lives have also boosted the high cost of health care and have generated wrenching moral and social questions. Our successes have created ethical and economic dilemmas. (Parsons, 1985, p. 466)

The Scarcity of Health Resources

Why we need to consider the allocation of resources in health care delivery is very simple. If we continue to use the resources at the rate that has become the norm in the past decade, soon there will not be enough to go around. To an uncomfortably large extent, health professionals themselves have been responsible for the growth of the problem by their understandable eagerness to use every available weapon in the arsenal to fight disease. While we may we believe that everyone has a right to health care, that right will become an empty one if we are unable to fulfil it because we lack the resources. In fact, in a number of situations, this crunch has already been felt. Unfortunately, although it is clear why we need to reconsider resource allocation, and it is easy to identify several contributing factors, how we ought to allocate is neither clear nor simple.

Overuse of Resources

First, doctors and allied health professionals have developed the habit of gambling on expensive, high-tech solutions, the efficacy of which has not always been tested adequately. The promotion of mammography is a good example of this phenomenon. Although the evidence of the efficacy, in the sense of longer survival rates, of this diagnostic procedure for low-risk women under age 50 has not been proven, some clinics and individual physicians continue to recommend it. Without evidence to prove its value, one can conclude that promotion of this procedure wastes time and resources. As critics of modern medical practice have said:

> In their desire to do everything possible to help their patients, doctors often succumb to the terrible pressure to take action…they jump the gun in advance of any good evidence to show their intervention will help, and wind up doing more harm than good, or wasting their time. (Rachlis and Kushner, 1989, p. 59)

It seems, then, that good intentions may have serious consequences in health care delivery, and thus do not provide a good enough basis for ethical decision making. As health professionals, we need to consider not only the individual patient (who may not even benefit from the treatment we have to offer), but also how many others might be denied treatment because of our decision to channel resources into areas that have so many unknowns. "As a society we are conditioned to the techno-logical fix—if we can do something, then we should do it, no matter the cost" (Seiden, 1985, p. 137).

The development of the artificial heart is a dramatic example of high-tech health care at its most controversial and complex. As resources are channelled into re-search, development, and testing of the artificial heart, those caregivers involved do not seem to have yet taken the time to consider what will actually happen should their work be successful. A high-incidence disease in North America, heart disease touches hundreds of thousands of lives. If this enormously expensive technology were available to all these people, the costs would be astronomical. Individuals would be saved from dying from a relatively acute illness only to develop more chronic and costly illnesses before they finally succumb. Will this technology only be available to the rich or, in a government-funded system, how will it be decided who will receive an artificial heart when we cannot afford to give one to everyone who could benefit? Perhaps we should not be using our hard-won resources in this way at all and should be looking for approaches that will be of benefit to larger numbers of people.

The second contribution we health professionals have made to the development of this problem of resource scarcity is our tendency to overuse services (Eisenberg and Rosoff, 1978). When health care services are used unnecessarily, other patients must either wait or do without. Fearing litigation, some caregivers tend to overuse diagnostic and therapeutic services in an attempt to avoid the possibility of patients claiming that everything available was not done. However, it is also clear that some of the blame for this overuse by caregivers can be attributed to patient demands for newer and more complex services, fuelled by reports in the popular press, as well as by health professionals themselves. Health care consumers see a news report about the new CT scanner in their local hospital and the next day begin demanding that this diagnostic tool be used every time they present with a headache. The use of diagnostic tests without medically valid indications threatens the integrity of the system and contributes to the abuse of available services. This problem may be more serious than we think. The caregiver must be able to inform patients about what they do and do not need. The extent to which the patient will heed this information is directly related to the amount of trust in the relationship.

Innovative technological advances themselves also need to be closely examined when considering best use of resources. Many new procedures, such as heart and liver transplantation or the use of artificial hearts, will only benefit small numbers of people. Questions concerning the good for the few vs. the good for the many are fundamental to the discussion of how we can ethically ration these scarce resources.

What Resources Are We Talking About?

Resources are those things that assist us in our goal to provide optimum health care. As resources are not necessarily tangible, we need to be aware of everything whose use needs to be monitored. In addition, we need to remember that none of the resources we use in health care delivery is limitless.

Money

The first resource that comes to mind is money. Health care costs money, and there is no doubt in anyone's mind today that spending must have limits. Health professionals, however, seem to think that bringing money into the discussion of clinical practice somehow degrades the noble work of health care and is therefore wrong. Most of us would agree that budgetary concerns provide a very poor basis for making diagnosis and treatment decisions, but, from a broader point of view, if money is never considered, it will surely run out.

Personnel and Equipment

Next, we need to be aware that personnel and equipment are limited, sometimes by money and sometimes by other factors. Because of availability of space, person-nel, and/or machinery, a hospital may only be able to run five renal dialysis ma-chines. Time, of course, being another finite resource, further restricts the number of patients who can be dialyzed in a week.

If we look specifically at personnel, certain geographic areas may be underserv-iced by medical specialists and particular allied health workers. A small community that does not have a resident physiotherapist, for example, cannot offer the same physical rehabilitative services as communities where physiotherapists are in greater supply. Thus, through no one's fault, the resource is rationed and everyone does not have equal access.

Drugs

There are other specific areas where resources are limited. Certain drugs are not readily available. So-called "orphan" drugs are required by so few individuals that less research money is put into testing them; some pharmaceutical companies refuse even to produce them because of their questionable profit margins.

Organ Transplants

Organ transplantation is another specific area with very limited resources. Here is a classic example of our inability to provide help (a transplant) to every patient who could potentially benefit from the procedure. We are severely limited by the lack of availability of donor organs. One way of solving this and other limited resource problems is to increase the availability of the resource. In the case of organ donation, organ procurement services across North America have been working toward that end for many years, with little in the way of positive outcome. Thus, we are still faced with the problem of allocating those resources ethically.

Money, personnel, equipment, beds, time, energy, and body parts are just a few of the resources that are, or should be, limited. Most of us realize that we cannot devote more than a specified portion of our national income to health care. If steps are not taken soon to curb costs and spending, health care expenditures will expand even more dramatically (Fried, 1977).

Principles of Fairness

There are many ways of viewing the distribution of resources in health care, and we need to examine some basic principles that can guide our decision making. Consider the following ways in which you might choose to make decisions as to which patient will have access to a particular service when everyone cannot have access and all under consideration could benefit.

Ability to Pay

First, we could decide that each person will receive a level of health care according to his/her ability to pay. Evidence that this is happening already can be seen in media reports of patients being turned away from hospitals because they do not have the money to pay for care. We also now see private money-raising drives to enable specific individuals to receive high-profile medical services like transplants. Obviously, this method of making decisions is not in agreement with our basic principle of beneficence, to do good. Surely, there must be a better way to decide.

Past Contributions

Another decision-making principle is based on the idea that each person should receive health care according to his/her past contributions to society. This would be helpful in situations where the candidates for the only available heart are, for example, a well-known university professor and a drifter. The obvious problem with this approach is the amount of subjective input required on the part of the decision makers. Who has the right to decide which person has made more of a contribution to society? What value scale could possibly be devised to rate behavior and provide a basis on which to make such a decision?

Potential Contribution

Instead of looking at past contributions to society, perhaps it would be more judicious to provide health care to each individual according to his/her potential contributions to society. Thus, people who are judged to be more likely to make a greater contribution to society in the future and therefore would have more utility to us should be entitled to the best that health care has to offer. This approach, however, suffers from the same problems of subjectivity or difficulty in judging as the previous one, although its utilitarian basis appeals to some people.

Place in Line

An apparently fairer approach, and one that is becoming increasingly popular, is to provide health services to individuals according to their place in line. In this approach, the need to make decisions is minimized, because each person who requires the scarce service simply waits in line until his/her turn. However, most health professionals are uneasy with this approach. They feel that it is inherently wrong to make patients wait who are known to be so ill that detrimental effects on their health are likely. In fact, by the time some patients reach the head of the line their health will have deteriorated to the extent that they now will require even more of the resources than they would have needed had they been treated earlier. Thus, this is not a completely satisfactory solution.

Patient Need

The solution that satisfies many health professionals is to provide health services to each person according to his/her need. This seems to fit with the reasons why most of us entered the health professions in the first place, the desire to help as best we can. Health care consumers have needs, and we have the skills and knowledge to provide them with what they need. On a humane level, and in the interests of optimum health care and fairness in its delivery, this seems to be the best approach to deciding who gets what. Unfortunately, the application of this principle, too, poses difficulties. Who should decide what it is that the patient needs and how do you decide between conflicting needs? It still does not guide us in those situations in which there simply is not enough to go around to fulfil everyone's needs.

In making reasonable decisions about rationing scarce resources, and rationing those resources that are not yet scarce but may well be in the future, we need to look at the application of a number of the basic principles already discussed.

As the problem of scarce resources is basically a social one, it seems reasonable to consider the good of society, versus the good of the individual patient. An appli-

Possible Principles of Fairness

- To each according to his/her ability to pay.

- To each according to his/her past contributions.

- To each according to his/her potential.

- To each according to his/her place in line.

- To each according to his/her need.

Figure 7.1.

cation of the basic principles of ethics that guide health care practice in other situations will assist us in making hard choices.

Consider first a full application of the principle of beneficence. The tradition represented by the Hippocratic Oath was a patient-centered one which failed to consider benefits to all parties, even those only indirectly affected (Veatch, 1986). Today's problems require a rethinking of the application of this principle. Extending the concept of beneficence to include a wider context can help us to decide what should be done. When access to medical treatment is being denied to particular individuals, an ethical rationale based on the principle of doing the most good for the largest number of people is, at the very least, a defensible position.

A Practical Attempt: The Oregon Solution

Most health professionals are aware that, in reality, rationing goes on in health care institutions every day, even if they are unwilling to admit it; this lack of openness about current activities is unfair to the consumers of health care. One group of people who stand out from the rest in admitting that they need to ration health services, and that they wish to do it as openly and equitably as possible, is the state legislature of Oregon. Their approach may not solve all the woes that beset the health care system, but it is worth examining to analyze the bases upon which these legislators are making difficult choices.

The Oregon scheme is based on the premise that the citizens of the state must have universal access to a basic level of care, which includes those health services that are considered to be most important and effective. It stresses that the system must be economically sustainable and that health care expenditures must be balanced with a number of other related areas (Kitzhaber, 1989). Once a price tag has been established for each service not considered basic and essential, these services are ranked by a Health Services Commission, which includes public input. The rankings depend on the proven clinical effectiveness of each service and the current social values attached to it (Silversides, 1990). Then, a package of services is drawn up, working down as far as the available money will go. The purpose is to design a medical delivery system which will do the greatest good for the greatest number of people, and to avoid spending vast sums of money on individual procedures that have very little hope of success.

By mid-1991, the Oregon legislature had ranked 709 medical services and drew the line at 587 services that would be financed under the concept of basic health services. These 587 services represented 90% of the cost of all the services ranked.

> Services provided under the standard benefit package encompass preventive care for children and adults, including dental care, treatment for accidents and injuries, immunizations, prenatal care, and treatment for life-threatening conditions. (Sipes-Metzler, 1991, p. 13)

Although not everyone agrees with this radical approach, it can only be considered radical because it has never been done before and because it is so painfully honest. But, can we fault the planners for honesty? On a philosophical level, it may be very easy to agree that this is a sane, moral, and humane approach; however, in reality, many members of the helping professions will have difficulty with this solution because "it is easier to say no to invisible people; it is much harder to say no to a person who has a face, a family, and a name" (Rooks, 1990, p. 43). On a day-to-day basis, our patients are anything but invisible.

The Oregon approach is the way of the future in health care delivery. Due consideration is given to the individual patient, but similar consideration is given to what the individual decision will mean in the larger context. For example, will agreeing to spend $100,000 on sending a very sick little child off to another state, province, or country to receive a treatment that is highly likely to be unsuccessful mean that thousands of unborn children are deprived of the best possible start because we cannot afford to give their mothers basic prenatal support? These are the kinds of considerations that must be taken into account by every modern health practitioner.

Summary: Fairness in Practice

As a person dedicated to giving care where it is needed, it may be anathema to you that economic considerations play even the smallest part in your clinical decision making. And certainly the realities of economic restraints should not be the only basis upon which we decide how to treat patients. We do, however, have to be sensitive to our social responsibilities.

Questions for Discussion and/or Review

1. What resources are now scarce or will soon be scarce if current rates of use continue or grow?

2. In your opinion, do health professionals overuse resources? In what way? Why? What results from this kind of use? Give examples from your experience to support your opinion.

3. What societal pressures lead to overuse of resources?

4. Have you dealt with any shortages in your job? What kind? How did they affect your work?

5. Identify the bases for deciding allocation of scarce resources. Which one(s) do you agree with? Why?

Recommended Reading

Leaf, Alexander. "The Doctor's Dilemma—and Society's Too," *New England Journal of Medicine*, 310 (March 15, 1984), 718–721.

Parsons, Arthur. "Allocating Health Care Resources: A Moral Dilemma," *Canadian Medical Association Journal*, 132 (February 15, 1985), 466–469.

Rooks, Judith P. "Let's Admit We Ration Health Care—Then Set Priorities," *American Journal of Nursing*, 90 (June, 1990), 39–43.

Part II

The Issues

8

High-Tech Medicine

In this chapter:

- ■ The nature and growth of high-tech medicine

- ■ Reasons for the growth of high-tech medicine
  - Scientific discoveries and inventions
  - Media reporting
  - Business promotion and marketing

- ■ Results of the growth of high-tech medicine
  - Increase in life expectancy
  - Increase in numbers of medical specialties
  - Increase in numbers of health professionals
  - Increased costs
  - Dehumanizing health care

- ■ Putting humanity back into health care

Science is a first-rate piece of furniture for a man's upper chamber, if he has common sense on the ground floor.

Oliver Wendell Holmes, 1872

This century has seen phenomenal advances in health care never dreamed of by the caregivers of almost 100 years ago. At the beginning of the twentieth century, the most that people could hope for from health care was to have their symptoms treated. If they broke bones, they could expect them to be set. If they had coughs, they might receive a poultice intended to alleviate some of the discomfort. Little thought was given to the possibility that a propensity to break bones might be related to an underlying disease process like osteoporosis or that a cough might signal lung cancer. Even if some people realized that there was more to the symptoms than met the eye, nothing could be done anyway. Medicine had little to offer, and patients expected nothing more. Indeed, the "laying on of hands," a traditional part of health care delivery, was almost all that could be offered, and it was highly regarded. Times have indeed changed.

No one wishes to return to the days when many deaths resulted from infectious diseases and the average life expectancy in North America did not exceed 50 or 55. Nevertheless, there is no denying that modern advances in medical technology have irreversibly altered the way that health care is delivered, not only from a scientific, but also from a humanistic point of view. Following in the wake of these extraordinary advances in technology are a whole host of difficult ethical dilemmas.

The Nature and Growth of High-Tech Medicine

High-technology medicine can be likened to a monster which, feeding on brilliant discoveries, medical egos, media attention, and the free enterprise system, has grown to such unwieldy proportions that it threatens to engulf us if we do not learn how to use it more wisely. But before we can discuss how to control this monster, we need to understand where it came from, how it grew so large, and how we have allowed it to dominate our professional practice.

The rapid growth of the monster would never have been possible, of course, without the truly amazing technological discoveries made in the past decades. Vastly improved surgical techniques, heart-lung machines, new drugs, organ replacements, reproductive interventions, CT scanners, nuclear magnetic resonance imaging, and many other new therapeutic or diagnostic tools have revolutionized the practice of medicine and the delivery of health care. As a result, modern medical technology has given health professionals enormous new powers. We have been granted the ability, to a significant extent, to exercise control over life and death. In a sense, the new technologies have given us the ability to play God.

Furthermore, hospitals today are quite different places from what they were even 30 years ago. Technology now plays such an important part in diagnostics and therapeutics, as well as in the computerized engineering and business administration systems, that patients often feel that the human element of their care has been severely minimized. Unfortunately, although the consumers of health care recognize that this is detrimental to the overall quality of the care they receive, some health professionals have succumbed to the lure of technology.

Many current nursing contracts, for example, provide extra pay to those nurses who work in intensive care units and other highly technological areas, such as recovery rooms and operating theatres. In our economically based society, these higher salaries imply higher regard for that kind of nursing. But, how can you compare the specialized skills and knowledge of the ICU nurse caring for her one or two critically ill patients with the knowledge and skills of the nurse caring for half a dozen cancer patients who are living through their final days or even hours? Is the nurse with technological expertise more valuable than the nurse with highly developed counseling skills who will assist many terminally ill people toward the kind of peaceful deaths impossible to achieve in intensive care? Unfortunately, the message sent to health professionals and society by higher monetary reward is that the person who is more technologically expert is more valuable.

This inequity of reward and the philosophy which sustains it is evident across North America, not only in nursing, but also in medicine. "Technique-oriented procedures receive greater compensation than do cognitive acts...the 'laying on of hands'" (James et al., 1990, p. 264). The "cutting specialities," i.e. surgeons, are usually at the higher end of the income scale, while psychiatrists and pediatricians bring up the rear. Financial incentives, then, may play a part not only in the selection of individual approaches to patient care, but even in the choice of specialties for new medical, nursing, and other graduates. The temptation to practise glamorous and highly paid high-tech medicine is hard to resist.

Another obvious result of this high-tech medicine monster is the proliferation of allied health professionals. For example, before the advent of open-heart surgery, specially trained perfusionists were not needed. Now, we see an enormous growth in the numbers of technical specialists, such as biomedical engineers, radiological technologists and their subspecialties, respiratory technologists, nuclear medicine technologists, ultrasonography technicians, dialysis technicians, and the list goes on. Indeed, each advance in medical technology brings with it new personnel requirements. Thus, fragmentation of care continues, costs creep ever skyward, and new groups are continually created who owe their jobs to the new high-tech medicine.

Of course, medical technology has not evolved to this point without some outside help as well. One of the most insidious contributing factors to the growth of this monster and the dilemmas that have surfaced with it is the media attention accorded to medical advances. Medically related stories make good copy, as the editors and reporters say, and good copy sells. A number of high-tech medical diagnostic and treatment approaches have captured the imagination of the media. As a result, such procedures as organ transplantation, cardiac surgery and MRI, and genetic engineering now have very high-profile status and are well known to the public.

As mentioned before, the media is the main source of health-related information for large numbers of North Americans. In their book, *Warning: The Media May be Harmful to Your Health*, Heussner and Salmon (1988) paint a very grim picture. Their premise is that the way medical information is communicated via the media is seriously flawed and "…lacks safeguards to protect the public from gullible reporters, entrepreneurial scientists, profit-minded medical manufacturers, and quacks…." (p. ix).

Another serious problem is that the media consumers lack knowledge of the issues to bring to their consumption of these medical stories. This lack of information and understanding on the part of the public leads them to believe that the so-called breakthroughs reported in the media immediately convert to new, readily available diagnostic or treatment modalities. Like the health care providers, they, too, are lured very easily into the belief that technologically oriented, quick-fix medicine is the best health care. Thus, fuelled by demand, the monster grows.

A final external factor that contributes to the growth of this high-tech medicine monster is the free enterprise market system. The marketing of medical equipment, supplies, and pharmaceuticals is big business in the US and Canada, and manufacturers of these goods have a vested interest in promoting their use, often at the expense of the solid research necessary to determine their efficacy. Owners of a private clinic, for example, may be enticed by the manufacturer to purchase the latest technological equipment and then find themselves forced to use this machinery on patients in order to pay for the initial outlay and the upkeep costs, sometimes with little indication that the patient really needs the procedure. In addition, media releases from the manufacturers, extoling the benefits of the product, increase public demand for expensive equipment.

At this point, the question to consider is whether technology is truly fulfilling our needs as a society, or we are fulfilling technology's needs. In other words, are we using technology for our objectives, or is the medical machine so out of hand that we are controlled by it? This is the crux of the ethical dilemmas posed by the issues that we will present in the following chapters.

There is no question that both health professionals and the public are becoming more and more concerned about this technological trap in which we find ourselves. In the fall of 1989, a conference called "Ethical Choices in the Age of Pervasive Technology" brought together over 800 attendees representing disciplines as diverse

Equation for Dehumanization of Health Care Delivery

Free Enterprise + technology + emotionalism

+

Increased demand for technological intervention

=

Increased costs to society
(economic, social)

+

Dehumanization of Health Care

Figure 8.1.

as medicine, law, labour, theology, the environment, to mention a few, all of whom were interested in discussion about how we might better manage the use of technology. Conspicuous by their absence, however, were the scientists, who apparently believed that the conference represented opposition to technological and scientific progress (Wiseman, 1989). What this conference did show, however, was that many segments of society are becoming concerned about where we are headed in the future and how we might get this monster under control to do the most good for the most people.

One of the results of the current love affair of health care with technology is the creation of a new kind of patient. These are the chronic patients who find only temporary reprieves from their ills with widely publicized high-tech treatment. While it is true that blame for the creation of these patients cannot be placed entirely on the shoulders of the caregivers (indeed, patient input is and must be taken into consideration), we must accept some responsibility for deceiving the public, for allowing them to believe in the unfailing abilities of high-tech medicine (Hutchison, 1988). High technology in health care is not infallible and has distinct limitations. Health professionals are responsible for knowing what these limitations are and for ensuring that patients, too, understand them.

The creation of these new chronic patients has led also to increased need for social support systems that are very expensive and not always available. Very ill patients who are maintained on dialysis, for example, create social and economic burdens to the system and have, at the very least, a questionable quality of life.

The equation presented in Figure 8.1 above summarizes the factors that are contributing to what critics of technological medicine have referred to as the dehumanization of health care delivery.

So, what do we do about it?

Putting Humanity Back into Health Care

As we will discuss in the next few chapters, high-tech medicine and the problems associated with it are here to stay. Future advances in medicine and health care delivery will present caregivers with more and different dilemmas. For example, who would have believed that, today, we would be considering the ethical and legal implications of ownership of frozen embryos? And yet this is only one of the many controversial issues currently being debated. We cannot know the exact nature of the issues of tomorrow, but given the urgency of the current situation and the future which looms ahead, we need to devise a way of thinking about these dilemmas so that some measure of humanity can be restored to our high technology medical world.

First, we need to recognize that the current concern for ethics in health care does not exist because we are more sensitive to morality than our predecessors. To tell the truth, it is the case that we are frightened of our abilities to control, to a significant degree, life and death. Practising in the era of high-tech health care delivery is an enormous responsibility, and each caregiver needs to scrutinize critically his/her own value systems and develop abilities to make moral decisions that consider not just the individual, but also the greater good.

Second, we need to keep technological innovation in perspective. We need always to ask the following questions in general, as well as in specific clinical situations:

- To what extent are the quality and quantity of the patient's life extended by the use of high-tech approaches?
- To what extent does a decision affecting a single patient also affect society at large? Future patients?
- What are the specific social outcomes of the treatment?
- Where is research in this particular technological area headed in the future?
- Are you as an individual caregiver impressed by the lure of high technology?
- Can you put yourself on the opposing side of the decision that first comes to your mind?

Obviously, the answers to these questions will not provide you with all you need in order to make decisions; there is no precise answer in ethics. But these and similar queries do provide you with a starting point for discussion with other health professionals who are also involved in the care of the patient and whose input is vital to a full hearing on these issues.

Summary

High technology in health care delivery is here to stay. Scientific research and development, along with profit-minded manufacturers of medical equipment and the ever-present mass media, have all played significant roles in the development of the high-tech approach which threatens to replace some of the more humanistic ways of relating to patients. However, the development of high-tech medicine has important positive aspects—we now live longer and healthier lives. As health professionals we must rethink our use of high technology so that we may begin to value more highly the art of compassion and caring that were the hallmarks of health care before machines came between us and our patients.

Questions for Discussion and/or Review

1. Prepare an argument for or against high-tech medicine and debate with someone who takes a position opposite to yours.
2. Research the origins of one new high-tech development in your field. What problems (if any) do you see in its current and future use?
3. Identify the factors that have contributed to the growth of high-tech medicine.
4. Identify some results of high-tech medicine. Divide them into two categories: beneficial and harmful.

Recommended Reading

Jacobson, Erika. "How To Ease the Ordeal," *American Journal of Nursing*, 90 (May, 1990), 40–42.

James, A.E., R.M. Zaner, J.E. Chapman, and C.L. Partain. "Technology and 'Turf': Medicine in Conflict," *Humane Medicine*, 6 (Autumn, 1990), 264–268.

Rakoff, Vivian. "The Fatal Question: Should the Irreversibly Ill be Kept Technically Alive?" *Saturday Night*, (May, 1985), 30–37.

9

Reproductive Technology

In this chapter:

■ Ethical issues arising from new
  reproductive technologies

- Reproductive enslavement

- Commodification of children

- Access to technology

- Mother vs. child: rights in conflict

■ Clinical issues arising from new
  reproductive technologies

- Infertility

- Sex preselection

- Embryo research

- Fetal therapy

*The basic evolutionary trends manifest in advanced industrial technology,
the longer life span and the increasing control of our biology insure that
the sex-role revolution which started as the women's movement will continue.*

Betty Friedan, *The Second Stage*, 1981

In the ethical minefield of modern medicine, there are full-fledged battles for su-
premacy going on at the two opposite ends of life—birth and death. Nowhere are
the issues more pressing and emotion-laden than in the specialties concerned with
bringing a new human being into the world and seeing one out. This chapter will
examine that first area, in which the new reproductive technologies, as we define
them here, encompass all those technological procedures that assist a human being
to conceive and carry another human being to be born into the world. Even in the
recent past, in the normal course of life, adult human beings either did or did not
engage in sexual intercourse, either did or did not have offspring, who either were
or were not normal, with a degree of control existing (and this, too, is arguable) only
in the first of these. Clearly, some people were not happy with the course of events
in their own lives, but little could be done about it. In today's world, where we seek
to control everything around us, the notion of leaving any of these processes to
chance seems as much of an anachronism as the chastity belt. Medical research and
the subsequent application of this research to the process of reproduction has
provided us with some of the control that we seek.

Sometimes it seems that the list of new medical technological innovations length-
ens with each passing day, and the list of reproductive technologies is no different.
Some of these new approaches include: in vitro fertilization; artificial insemination;
cryopreservation of eggs, sperm and preembryos; uterine lavage for preembryo
transfer; and research on preembryos.

What Are the Ethical Problems in Reproductive Medicine?

At first glance, it may appear that any innovation providing us with more control
over our reproduction and thus our lives and happiness must also contribute to the
expansion of our freedom as human beings. Why, then, is there so much heated
debate in this area both inside and outside the health professions? Some of the
serious ethical problems spawned by the new reproductive technologies include:
actual and potential effects of these technologies on women and children; the potential for further commodification of children; inequality of access; the rights of the
fetus; embryo research; the conflicting rights of women and their offspring; and the
potential, overall effects on society.

Reproductive Slavery

Although males and females are both intimately involved in the normal processes of reproduction, the array of technological approaches available and the physical and social problems they are designed to solve lead us to the conclusion that any discussion of reproductive technology is, to a significant degree, a women's issue.

Aside from the specific concerns inherent in the clinical approaches that we will discuss later, an increasing body of opinion now believes that the new reproductive choices do not lead to more freedom but to a form of reproductive slavery for women. This viewpoint is argued cogently in current feminist literature. Since prenatal sex identification has become possible as a by-product of some forms of prenatal diagnosis, the argument suggests that if male offspring were encouraged and female offspring discouraged by means of terminating pregnancies of female fetuses, the proportion of females in the population might drop so low that women would become prized for their reproductive function and be forced to reproduce.

Commodification of Children

Reproductive control can further the commodification of children. Children are becoming more valuable, not for themselves as individuals, but for what they can add to their parents' lives, much like a flashy car or an expensive house.

Joan Rothschild, professor of political science at the University of Lowell, Massachusetts, believes that one of the most insidious consequences of the new reproductive technologies is the movement toward increasing selectivity and thus the engineering of the "perfect" child, an endpoint that will have dramatic consequences for society (Rothschild, 1991).

Rothschild concludes that new technological advances like prenatal screening, genetic engineering, in vitro fertilization, sex preselection, fetal therapy, and selective abortion provide us with such control that, in many cases, we can now prevent the "imperfect" child from ever being born. The definition of perfection is unclear, but such techniques do suggest an intolerance for those human beings with less utility to society. In addition, if true, this conclusion furthers the argument that medical technology and those who offer it to patients are more concerned about medical cultural goals of disease prevention and patient autonomy than about public interest and the future good of society.

Inequality of Access

Typically, the North American patient who has access and makes use of the new reproductive technologies is white, upper middle class, and has less tolerance for handicapped children than those of lesser means and minority extraction (Rothschild, 1991).

Summary of Ethical Problems in the Application of the Reproductive Technologies

- Effects of technology on reproductive freedom

- Increasing commodification of children

- Fetal rights

- Conflict of rights: mother vs. fetus

- Access to scarce resources

- Engineering of perfection

Figure 9.1.

One striking and worrisome social consequence of this privileged access may be the clustering of "imperfect" children, and subsequent clustering of "imperfect" adults, in the lower socio-economic groups in the community. The demands for social support systems in the future to deal with their problems could be enormous.

Mother vs. Child: Rights in Conflict

As we have already discussed, modern history has seen the emergence of a variety of "rights" movements, among the most recent of which is the fetal rights movement. This concern for the rights of the unborn is the direct result of modern technological innovation.

The twentieth week of gestation has often been suggested as the critical point of fetal viability. This scientific benchmark can be used to determine when the fetus should be treated as a patient on its own. However, continuing advances in neonatology constantly push the age of viability earlier and earlier, and universal agreement has yet to be achieved on this question, as on so many others.

Recent legal opinions reflect a shift from the concept that the fetus is an integral part of the pregnant woman toward the concept that the fetus has rights on its own (Johnsen, 1987). This expansion of fetal rights seems to limit directly the rights of the pregnant woman. For example, what obligations does the pregnant woman have toward her unborn child? Is the pregnant woman who takes cocaine, drinks alcohol excessively, smokes heavily, or otherwise puts her unborn child at risk legally liable? There have been some reported cases of women being arrested and charged with offences of harming their unborn children by not providing adequate prenatal care. And yet, despite this kind of infringement of individual rights, it is clear that improved prenatal care can add to the greater good, as healthier babies will result. Thus the argument that society's rights need to be considered may help in reaching conclusions. This, of course, gives rise to the further question of whether society should finance a high standard of prenatal care for those who cannot afford it, and if so, how.

Making Ethical Judgments

Even slight knowledge of the available technological innovations in reproductive medicine leaves the impression that the objectives of those involved in their development is to provide access to a perfect baby, at the perfect time, for every person who wants one. To analyze this idea and where it is leading us, we need to examine and understand both the ethical and the specific clinical issues and determine whose rights we, as health professionals, need to uphold, and which principles ought to provide us with guidance.

Several years ago, the Ethics Committee of the American Fertility Society examined the ethical concerns arising from these new reproductive technologies. This committee concluded that there are four major areas that health professionals and patients must consider in making an ethical judgment about these technologies:

- the degree of artificiality of the new reproductive technology;
- the moral status of the human preembryo;
- the role of the family or genetic lineage;
- the appropriate role of government (American Fertility Society, 1986, p. 76S).

Obviously, these considerations do not provide any clear framework for ethical decision making in this area as there is no general agreement on some of their basic premises. For example, there is no clear-cut way to determine the relative degree of artificiality of one technological approach over another. Second, although a human preembryo is defined as the stage before the rudiment of the person appears in the second week after fertilization, and the stand has been taken that this entity is different from an embryo, there is no general agreement about its moral status yet.

These are some of the ethical problem areas that we need to keep in mind as we examine the clinical issues and the possible consequences of each.

Specific Clinical Issues

The reasons why adult human beings want to have children have never been precisely identified. Ask a dozen couples (or individuals) why they want a child or

> ## Clinical Issues in Reproductive Technology Resulting in Ethical Dilemmas
>
> - Infertility
>
> - Sex preselection
>
> - Embryo research
>
> - Fetal therapy
>
> *Figure 9.2.*

have a child and a dozen different responses are given. The fact remains that procreation is one of the goals of human beings.

Infertility

The first and most pervasive current clinical issue in current reproductive technology is infertility. Individuals and couples who realize that they are unable to have a child in the normal way react with a variety of emotions, from shock, to anger, to denial. As recently as 30 years ago, their only recourse was adoption. But reproductive technology has changed all that.

Infertility has risen dramatically in the past 25 years. In the usually most fertile age group of women, 20 to 24 years, infertility rose 177% between 1965 and 1982 (Wallis, 1984). Among the probable causes of this increase are the sequelae of sexually transmitted diseases, abortion, and contraceptive devices. The emotional impact of this infertility is devastating, and thus the demand for solutions has come not only from the health professions, but from consumers themselves. One infertility counselor has described the impact as follows:

> Infertility rips at the core of the couple's relationship; it affects sexuality, self-image and self-esteem. It stalls careers, devastates savings, and damages associations with friends and family. (Wallis, 1984, p. 40)

Modern medical technology offers several approaches to solve this problem of childlessness, with varying degrees of success. These approaches include artificial insemination by donor sperm when the problem can be attributed completely to the father, and a variety of permutations and combinations of donor sperm and eggs, in vitro fertilization, and surrogate mothers, based on the degree of incapacity of the mother and/or father. There are ethical questions concerning these procedures themselves, as well as concerns about where they are leading us. In addition, there are knotty legal problems in separating the rights of the biological family from the rights of the social family, all the while considering that the child conceived in artificial ways has rights as well. There are potentially eight individuals who could claim legal rights to the child, depending upon the exact nature of the coupling which resulted in the fertilized ovum, i.e. a sperm donor, his wife, the egg donor, her husband, the surrogate, her husband, and the mother or the father for whom the child was conceived.

The potential for expanded uses of the available technology to treat infertility requires us, as health professionals, to consider these issues of outcomes and rights with an emphasis on making the best decision not only for the individual patient, but also for the greater good. Consider the following questions:

- If it is ethical to use artificial insemination to facilitate conception when the male is infertile, is it ethical to use artificial insemination to assist in the engineering of the "perfect" child (as alluded to earlier in this chapter)?
- If it is ethical to recover eggs for in vitro fertilization, is it also ethical to remove eggs for research purposes? If so, which ones? Perhaps those fertilized for this specific purpose? What makes these two scenarios different?
- If it is ethical for surrogate mothers to be used to assist childless couples to have children, can this service be extended to a woman who does not want to interrupt her career to have a child? Would this provide a valuable service or institute a form of prostitution?
- Is the media hype surrounding the successes of new technologies causing undue hardship for vulnerable people who will do almost anything to conceive?

We do not yet know the right answers to these questions. As health professionals are the ones who carry out these procedures, we need to consider where the technology is leading us.

Sex Preselection

The second clinical issue in reproductive technology is sex preselection. The number and precision of the new technologies in prenatal diagnosis have afforded us the ability to determine the sex of the fetus, sometimes long before birth. Ultrasound is capable of giving us this information, as is amniocentesis and the newest and earliest approach to prenatal diagnosis, chorionic villus sampling.

Sex preselection is an especially troubling ethical issue for health professionals, primarily because, at the present time, the actual selection of the sex of a child can only be achieved by selective abortion, i.e. by aborting the unwanted sex. Apart from strictly medical grounds for selective abortion presented in such cases as the carrying of sex-linked diseases, a considerable body of opinion holds that both moral and social arguments weigh heavily against the use of the tools of prenatal sex determination for sex selection. Wertz and Fletcher (1989) present three societal arguments against sex preselection by any means. These include the need to avoid:

- unbalancing the sex ratio;
- diminishing the status of women (assuming the sex preference would be for males);
- unbalancing the birth order with its psychological and legal ramifications if, for example, most families acted upon their preference for firstborn boys (p. 23).

On the other hand, some people suggest that ensuring the desired gender for off-spring results in happier family arrangements and thus happier children. There has been, however, a well-documented preference for male offspring, particularly when the family is to consist of only one child, and thus we could anticipate that the gender balance could change drastically.

This issue raises a number of questions for consideration:

- Is sex selection, based as it usually is upon a preference for one sex over the other, sexist?
- Is it ethical to perform abortions to accommodate the sex preferences of some cultures?
- Is it ethical to use costly, limited medical resources for nonmedical reasons when women who need prenatal diagnostic facilities for medical reasons may not have access to them?

It is particularly important to apply the principle of fairness in grappling with these questions, particularly the last one. The increasing use of scarce and often costly medical resources to deal not with medical problems, but rather with non-medical, social ones, is of grave concern to all those health professionals and members of the public who recognize that the resources are not infinite. It is not yet clear to us where the developments in reproductive technology are leading, but we ought to take a proactive approach in meeting the future, rather than a reactive one.

Embryo Research

Another important clinical issue of reproductive technology is embryo research. Many of the current techniques (e.g. in vitro fertilization) present us with what could be considered extra embryos. Researchers often face the decision to either destroy the extras, or possibly use them more advantageously—that is, as research subjects. Several issues arise from this latter practice.

First is the problem of consent. It is unclear whether the individuals who provided the eggs and sperm to produce these embryos should have rights. They can hardly be called "parents" in this context. The real issue here is the actual status of the embryo, which is also unclear, both legally and ethically at this time.

Second is the problem of when to stop nurturing an embryo should the decision be made that it is ethical to conduct research on it. As we gain more and more precise information about how an embryo's nervous system and brain develop, interest is growing in developing a definition of brain birth to signal the beginning of life (just as we have new, more precise ways of determining death, using brain death criteria). A recent medical discussion paper on fetal rights indicates a belief that a fetus becomes a person when the nervous system "has developed to the point where it meets the basic requirements for sapient cognitive awareness irrespective of its level of sophistication" (Sullivan, 1990, p. 404). Similarly, the American Fertility Society has determined that up until about the fourteenth day, when the primitive streak, the anlage of the neural tube, appears, experimentation on human embryos is permissible (Hill, 1986).

Even with these guidelines, we need to consider the following questions:

- Is it ethical to conduct research on leftover embryos?
- Is it ethical to waste them?
- Do the donors of the eggs and sperm that produce the embryos have any rights, or the only rights, regarding their disposal?

Fetal Therapy

The last significant problem that we would like to consider is fetal therapy. Each year the number of congenital defects that can be treated in the womb increases. New diagnostic modalities such as ultrasound, amniocentesis, fetoscopy, and amniography, which all afford the opportunity to diagnose these abnormalities prenatally, have led to increasing interest and advantage in treating the baby prenatally.

However, the ethical conflicts in this area are complex. First, there is a distinct ideological clash between the belief in the right of women to have free choice of abortion and the concept of the unborn child as a person who should have access to treatment for abnormalities. If we do consider the fetus to be a person with rights, clearly, a major conflict can develop between the rights of the fetus and the rights of the mother. As medical technology concentrates more and more on the fetus, the mother becomes secondary and, in these instances, may become valuable only as the environment or repository for the developing child. The possibility of this rights conflict is one of the major areas of future concern in reproductive technology and needs to be considered in some detail.

Summary

Advances in reproductive technology have created enormous ethical dilemmas, and as the technology improves, the morass becomes deeper. All health professionals involved in any aspect of this technological revolution need to consider their own values when assisting the health care community and its consumers to make salient decisions.

Questions for Discussion and/or Review

1. Should we ever interfere in the reproductive process? Give reasons for your answer.

2. Which reproductive technologies are acceptable to you? How do you justify them? Which are not acceptable to you? Why do you reject them?

3. Choose one form of reproductive technology and discuss the ethical problems it creates.

4. The question of surrogacy has been widely debated. What advantages and disadvantages do you see in this practice? Use actual reported examples to support your arguments if you can.

5. What choices would you present to an infertile couple who are investigating the available possibilities? What techniques (if any) would you recommend? What techniques (if any) would you not recommend?

6. Do you agree that the use of some of the new technologies in this area constitutes a form of slavery for women? Discuss and support your arguments with ethical principles.

7. Should health care workers ever be free to refuse to participate in a procedure that is against their moral beliefs?

8. What limits (if any) should be placed on the use of human eggs, sperm, or fetal tissue?

Recommended Reading

Johnsen, Dawn. "A New Threat to Pregnant Women's Autonomy," *Hastings Center Report*, 17 (August, 1987), 33–40.

Wallis, Claudia. "The New Origins of Life," *Time*, (September 10, 1984), 40, 42–44, 49, 51.

Wertz, Dorothy & John Fletcher. "Fatal Knowledge? Prenatal Diagnosis and Sex Selection," *Hastings Center Report*, 19 (May-June, 1989), 21–27.

10

The Neonatal Intensive Care Dilemma

In this chapter:

- ■ The decision to treat

- ■ Who should make the decisions to provide, not provide, or withdraw care

- ■ Guidelines for assessing quality of life

- ■ How to allocate scarce resources
  - The triage solution
  - The first-come/first-served solution
  - The alternative priority rule

Every baby has its chance.

A neonatal I.C.U. nurse

There may be no other area of health care where recent technological advances arouse such overpowering emotions as in the intensive medical treatment of infants who have had the misfortune of being born prematurely, with congenital anomalies or diseases. In cemeteries across North America the many tombstones proclaiming the burial of the "infant son of" or the "infant daughter of" are evidence that early death was a commonplace phenomenon in the past. Today, with the dramatic improvement in our ability to treat sick babies, particularly in the past three decades, the loss of an infant child is rare indeed.

As techniques for dealing with very sick adults improved, techniques then became available on experimental bases for application to increasingly smaller, sicker, and more impaired neonates. As a result, many babies who formerly died now survive. By 1975, neonatology had become a Board Certified specialty in the United States. By 1986, it became an accredited subspecialty, without certification in Canada.

The whole story, however, has not been idyllic. As in most other areas of technological advance in health care, the application of new diagnostic and treatment modalities to sicker babies, those who might have been previously labelled with the imprecise term, "nonviable," have had their critics. They began asking a seemingly simple question: Are we doing more harm than good? The term "harm," in this case, must be defined broadly enough to encompass the following considerations:

- iatrogenic complications;
- family distress;
- poor quality of life;
- financial burdens to society.

The ethical issues we face today in neonatology are products of a system that has unreservedly supported technological advances. Although health professionals seem to resent the suggestion that they are playing God, it is no longer possible to avoid doing so, because of the simple availability of the technology (Fost, 1981). Even a decision *not* to make use of those technological marvels is a God-like decision. Thus, the first hard question is how we are to decide on whether or not to institute treatment—which involves facing the underlying question of quality vs. quantity of life. Second, we must face the broader question of the accessibility to and allocation of scarce resources.

Whenever a baby is labelled "nonviable," "hopelessly ill," "terminally ill," "incurably ill," or any other such ambiguous classification, we set ourselves up for a chain reaction of preconceived notions about how we ought to behave toward that child. Thus we need to stay away from these labels and discuss each case in the context of the ethical principles that ought to guide our care each day of our professional lives.

Decisions: Whose Right, Whose Responsibility?

Health care delivery in neonatal intensive care faces two difficult ethical concerns: when to provide care and who should make the decision to provide (or not provide) care.

In other words, the three basic decisions that have to be made are:

- when to treat;
- when not to treat;
- when to stop treatment.

Likewise, there are three possible parties who have interests, responsibilities, and rights in making those decisions:

- health professionals, who may from time to time be represented by institutional ethics committees;
- parents;
- society, as represented by government.

How to Decide When to Treat: Some Guidelines

Fost (1981) identifies two basic presumptions that can justify decisions to treat, not to treat, or to stop treating:

- There is a generally shared presumption in western society that human life should be preserved, as is reflected in our laws, customs, and religious beliefs. The ethical principle of the sanctity of life underlies this presumption.
- However, it is becoming increasingly acceptable to propose that not everyone should have to continue to live. This assertion is based on the belief that individual human beings have a right to a minimum level of quality of life and should not have treatment forced on them if this minimum cannot be met. In addition, it is held that others who might benefit more should then have the right to the resources that might otherwise be wasted on those who will almost certainly soon die.

In the late 1970s, over 450 pediatricians and pediatric surgeons who were in positions to make treatment decisions for very sick neonates were surveyed for their opinions on how these decisions should be made. The majority of the respondents believed that not every infant's life should be maintained by the use of advanced technology and that this decision must be based on the best guess, from a medical point of view, about quantity and quality of life. They believed that these decisions should be made on a case-by-case basis and that parents, supported by physicians, should have both the right and the responsibility to make treatment decisions (Haslam, 1977).

In November 1983, a coalition of American organizations concerned with treatment of disabled babies issued a statement of principles to guide parents, doctors, governments, and other involved parties in making decisions about treatment (O'Neill, 1983). These principles indicated that:

- When medical care is clearly beneficial, it should always be provided, and a person's disability should never be the basis upon which a decision to withhold treatment is made.
- Once a decision has been made to treat, both government and private agencies have a responsibility to allocate sufficient resources for as long as is needed.
- More information about available resources for care of the disabled is needed by both parents and health professionals before decisions about treatment can be made.

At the time these principles were signed, one of the signatories, the Down's Syndrome Congress, headquartered in Chicago, issued a press release which stated: "...the National Down's Syndrome Congress supports and demands each person's inherent civil, human and legal rights earned by virtue of their birth. All have a 'potential' at birth that can only be fully realized according to opportunities offered during life."

The press release issued by the American Academy of Pediatrics, one of the hosts of the signing event, included comments by Dr. Paul Weherle, the president of the academy: "Some urgent issues remain to be resolved but these principles publicly reaffirm the sensitivity each of us shares in searching for fair and just solutions."

By 1984, the American Academy of Pediatrics' Infant Bioethics Task Force and Consultants issued "Guidelines for Infant Bioethics Committees" and in it recommended "that parents and physicians consult with an institutional ethics committee when decisions are contemplated to forego life-sustaining treatment" (Infant Bioethics Task Force, 1984). This recommendation was based on the belief that it was congruent with the conclusions of the President's Commission for the Study of Ethical Problems in Medicine, as well as research that had resulted in the 1983 report "Deciding to Forego Life-Sustaining Treatment."

In the 1990s, we have some direction, as well as some protection under the law.

> In the United States federal laws require doctors to begin treatment of all babies except those who would clearly not benefit. However, no regulations guide a physician's decision to stop treatment once it has been initiated. This has become a complex issue, as the very technology that saves babies also sometimes causes handicaps. (Schiff, 1990, p. 2)

The Problem of Definition: "Quality of Life"

If we accept that, in the North America of the 1990s, we are at least as concerned about quality as we are about quantity of life, perhaps even more so, then dilemmas about when to treat or not to treat sick babies become more a problem of definition of quality of life, a definition that remains elusive. In addition, we face the problem of defending any such definition against legal proceedings initiated by those who believe in the sanctity of life, regardless of its quality.

Daniel Callahan, Director of the Hastings Center, proposes that some degree of consistency in judgment and action is essential, and that the medical position should avoid the extreme views of either sanctity of life or quality of life (Gilmore, 1984). Again, however, to define precisely what constitutes quality seems an impossible quest, but there is some agreement that it ought to include consideration of the individual's physical, mental, and spiritual dimensions.

One quality of life index that has been proposed for adults provides an evaluation that is correct at any given point in time. It includes a quick assessment of:

- activity level—the degree of ability to get around;
- activities of daily living—ability to care for self;
- general health—including symptom control;
- support—significant others to do things with and for;
- outlook—including mood and the spiritual dimension.

On a scale of 0—2 for each item, the individual is assessed (Gilmore, 1984). A similar scale, using projected potential of an infant where possible, combined with the benefit/burden concept of treatment outcomes, can be a very useful tool for assessing the quality of a sick baby's life.

Who Makes the Decision?

Another difficult problem in dealing with babies, however, is the fact that adults must make this kind of decision for the child. In situations where the hopelessly ill patient is an adult, it is generally accepted that the patient him/herself will have important input into any decisions that will affect his/her life, insofar as it is possible to have that input. When the patient is a neonate, there can be no input from the individual patient, and therefore the issues are complicated further by having third parties make decisions.

Clearly, parents, health professionals, and, in some instances, institutional ethics committees have roles to play in making thorny decisions about treatment, non-treatment, and stopping treatment in sick neonates. These individual decisions can be assisted by the application of the basic principles of doing good and doing no harm. The role of society and/or government, however, is less clear, but until some general consensus is reached, outside party involvement from the judicial system should be expected.

When Resources Are Scarce: Being Just

Two realities must be kept in mind when discussing ethical dilemmas created by technological innovation. First, all resources are limited, although not all to the same extent; and second, supplying high technology health care results in increased expectations and demand. In the area of neonatal intensive care these factors raise two major questions for consideration:

- How do we decide which baby should be treated when there are not enough current resources for all to be treated?
- To what extent should limited, costly resources be used to treat very sick babies who have little hope of a normal life when that money might better be spent on services for optimizing the health and well-being of children with more potential?

Who Do We Treat? How Do We Decide?

Before we discuss each of these questions individually, it is important to recognize our responsibility in the dilemmas they pose. Health professionals are at the interface between the health care delivery system with its high-tech innovations and a society that is more and more distrustful and, at the same time, increasingly demanding. If we decide that the issues in resource allocation are too burdensome for us to make, then we have relinquished our responsibility, and the decisions will be made by others. While playing "gate-keeper" for the system may not be to your liking, innovation has made it an inevitable role of the modern caregiver, whose input is crucial to the development of a workable system. Those others to whom the decisions are otherwise abdicated may be outside agencies and/or governments, whose primary concern will be cost containment, not care of the individual patient (Schiff, 1990).

The Triage Solution

Dorland's Medical Dictionary (1965) defines triage as: "the sorting out and classification of casualties of war or other disaster, to determine priority of need and proper place of treatment" (p. 1610). There is little doubt in the minds of the parents of an infant with a serious medical problem and the health professionals that care for that neonate that a disaster has occurred. Thus, it seems appropriate that if decisions have to be made about which baby to treat when there clearly are not enough resources (e.g. neonatal intensive care beds) to treat all of them, principles of triage might be helpful in determining a just solution.

Triage systems are based on the utilitarian ethic of doing the most good for the greatest number—the application of which frequently relies on an assessment of social utility. Individuals may be given preference in treatment because of their perceived value to the community.

"Because it is impossible to treat all infants in need, preference should be given to those with the greatest hope of surviving with maximal function" (Johnsen and Garland, as quoted in Childress, 1983).

The First-Come/First-Served Solution

Another possible solution to this dilemma is to provide care solely on a first-come/first-served basis. Medical services are provided to all babies who need them, as soon as they are born, until the resources are exhausted.

Alternative Priority Rule

Childress (1983) proposes an "Alternative Priority Rule":

> ...if it is not possible to provide intensive care for all newborns when they need it in order to survive and when survival and intensive care would be in their best interests, priority should be determined by randomization or queuing unless there are major differences in their probabilities of survival. (p. 557)

In cases where decisions about who will be treated are necessary, the following assumptions underlie the application of the priority rule:

- There is clearly insufficient care to go around.
- Decisions are made to exclude those babies who are irreversibly dying.
- It is legitimate to make judgments that are in the best interests of the newborn.
- The parents and the caregivers are able to balance the benefits and the burdens to the child.

Obviously, not everyone will agree with these assumptions, but they do provide some guidance. If, after these concerns are answered, there are still babies whose needs cannot all be met, queuing is the suggested method. Thus, each case is judged independently from the others. This notion of independent judgment seems to have some rationale in the concept of justice.

Using Resources Wisely

The second question we must try to address concerns the extent to which it is appropriate to channel costly and limited resources into treatment for very sick babies who have little hope for a normal life, when that money might be better spent optimizing the health and well-being of children with more potential. In fact, it could be argued that money might even be better spent on preventative prenatal programs to avoid some of the congenital problems in the first place. This second question is very difficult to answer because, once again, it pits the needs of the individual against the needs of society.

A further complicating problem is the fact that making ethical decisions based on economic concerns for the greater good cannot guarantee that the funds *not* used to treat these particular babies will, indeed, find their way into the programs that, as health professionals, we believe are ethically more sound. Past experience with this reallocation argument (e.g. during the Vietnam war) suggests that the liberated funds will enter the same marketplace as all revenues and are as likely to end up in highway construction as in health (Fost, 1981, p. 19). The people currently charged with making such treatment decisions at the bedside are not the same people who will ultimately determine where health care dollars actually will be spent.

As there is no guarantee that, based on medical and ethical grounds, the greater good will be served, this argument is used by those health professionals who wish to abdicate any responsibility in making decisions about allocation of scarce resources on the macro level. They fear that money saved in any particular health care area will ultimately be channelled out of the health care system and thus see no point in making difficult decisions.

An even more basic problem concerns whether or not health professionals ought to be placed at all in the position of making these kinds of decisions that will affect society at large. Do health professionals have the ability to make such decisions and are they the most appropriate people to make them? There is much controversy about the answer to these questions. Some caregivers believe that they are neither competent nor authorized by society to make such decisions (Fost, 1981). Others believe just the opposite—that, although society at large ought to be making these decisions, the health care team should be providing concrete direction (Childress, 1983; Schiff, 1990). In spite of our general lack of expertise with economics, we are the ones with the expertise in health care.

Summary

Twentieth-century medical technology has enormously decreased infant morbidity and mortality, but at the same time has created new medical problems and a whole host of ethical dilemmas. Unfortunately, as technology in this area continues to advance, our ability to make salient ethical decisions continues to lag behind. We face more questions instead of more answers.

Questions for Discussion and/or Review

1. In your view, should attempts be made to save the lives of all newborns, without exception? On what principle(s) do you base your response?

2. How would you respond to parents who wish neonatal treatment continued that in your opinion will not be successful and is causing undue suffering?

3. Who should make the decisions about neonatal treatment?

4. When faced with scarce resources in neonatal care, on what basis do you think they should be allocated? Support your answer with specific reasons.

5. Discuss what "quality of life" means in the case of very young babies. Is it possible to balance the belief in the sanctity of life with a concern for quality of life?

Recommended Reading

Childress, James F. "Triage in Neonatal Intensive Care: The Limitations of a Metaphor," *Virginia Law Review*, 69 (1983), 547–561.

Fost, Norman. "Ethical Issues in the Treatment of Critically Ill Newborns," *Pediatric Annals*, 10 (October 10, 1981), 16–21.

Gilmore, Anne. "Sanctity of Life vs. Quality of Life—The Continuing Debate," *Canadian Medical Association Journal*, 130 (January 15, 1984), 180–181.

11

Organ Replacement Technology

In this chapter:

- ■ Development of organ replacement technology

- ■ Problems in the application of organ replacement technology
  - Lack of donors
  - Obtaining consent
- ■ Issues in organ replacement technology
  - Use of living donors
  - Use of anencephalic donors
  - Use of fetal tissue
  - Media attention and intervention
  - Allocating organs

It is easy to play the role of "savior" and preach the beatitude of high-tech medicine: Blessed are they whose organs have failed, for they shall receive a transplant.

Rosemary Hutchison M.D., C.C.F.P. in *Humane Medicine*, November, 1988

In 1984, Colorado Democratic Governor Richard Lamm created a furore when he was quoted as saying "…we've got a duty to die and get out of the way with all of our machines and artificial hearts, so that our kids can build a reasonable life" (Friedrich, 1984, p. 42). Although his sentiments are not shared by many health professionals in the field of organ transplantation, his viewpoint has some appeal and support.

The dramatic achievements in organ transplantation have made it one of the best publicized and well known of the new medical technologies. Advances in this area have enabled those whose bodies are wearing out naturally or are being destroyed by disease to live longer, more productive lives. Many survive who formerly would have died. However, organ transplantation presents us with many of the same ethical problems of other new specialties, as well as some unique dilemmas.

The History of Organ Transplantation

The practice of transplantation has been around for a very long time. References to the first blood transfusion, which is a tissue transplant in itself, can be found in medical histories of the fifteenth century. At that time there was also interest in the transplantation of teeth. Modern transplantation, however, is another product of the technological innovations of the twentieth century.

Although pioneers in the field attempted to transplant organs as early as 1902, their lack of knowledge about the immunological implications of exposing an individual to foreign antigens doomed those attempts to failure. The first successful kidney transplant reported in the medical literature was carried out in Boston in 1954. This attempt succeeded because the identical twin of the recipient was used as the live donor. With identical genetic material, the transplant worked.

Much of the research for the next three decades focused on the development of clinically useful immunosuppressive agents to solve the problem of rejection. At the same time, surgical techniques were improved. Finally, following the discovery and subsequent clinical introduction of Cyclosporin A, transplantation came of age in the 1980s, with increasing success. Today, it is possible to graft successfully a variety of organs, including kidneys (which are the most widely transplanted organ throughout the world), hearts, livers, pancreases, parts of the gastrointestinal system, lungs, skin, and a variety of tissues, including bone marrow and corneas.

The average citizen regards transplantation as a dramatic and awe-inspiring procedure, partially because of media exposure. Images of doctors, nurses, and technicians jetting from one part of the continent to another to harvest and then transplant organs would seem, at first glance, to be the stuff of fiction, but these scenarios are an everyday reality for some health professionals. The high-profile nature of the field contributes in no small measure to the many ethical problems that continue to plague transplant facilities. We will discuss some of the most pressing concerns that are unique to the field.

Organ Donor Problems

Without a doubt, the lack of organ donors leads to the most troubling moral dilemmas that face North American transplant facilities. As transplantation has become the treatment of choice for an increasing number of patients with end-stage organ failure, the main stumbling block to accessibility to these programs has been this scarcity of donor organs. As a result, transplant centers need to increase the number of organs available and to ration those that are available. The practices resulting from both these needs have spawned ethical problems.

Lack of Donors

Only about 2% of all individuals who die in North America in any given year die in such a way that they are suitable to donate organs for transplant. That is: the patient must die in a hospital from significant brain injury so that brain death criteria may be applied; the patient must have a stable pulse and blood pressure maintained artificially and have no history of significant medical problems in the past, including cancer or current systemic infection. Theoretically, in spite of these stringent criteria, if all potential donors could be converted into actual donors, more organs than are needed would be available. Where does the system break down?

The Issue of Consent

The main problem lies in obtaining consent. Many families do not wish to give consent, and health professionals may not ask for that consent. Although many opinion polls conducted in North America on the subject of organ donation indicate that most people are favorably disposed to the practice, the main reason that they or suitable family members do not become organ donors is because they either have not thought about it at all or are frightened at the thought.

> One objection to organ donation is the fear that the organs may be removed while we are still alive. The concept has surfaced in enough Edgar Allan Poe-type horror stories to make the most stalwart soul nervous. No matter how objectively one views the concept of brain death,

there is still something eerie to most people in the removal of a beating heart from a warm, albeit artificially breathing body. (Houlihan, 1988)

Other fears also play a part in hesitation about or rejection of the organ donation process. These include a fear of post-death bodily mutilation and the fear of death itself. For their part, health professionals find asking for organ donation one of the hardest requests to make.

For example, consider facing a distraught family that has just learned that their daughter, lying in an intensive care unit bed after an auto accident, is being tested for brain death determination. They look at her and, in spite of the equipment and lights and noises surrounding her in her cubicle, she seems to be only sleeping, and they remember her excitement about going to the school dance less than three hours earlier. They have hardly had time to assimilate your uncomfortable words indicating death when you realize that now is the time you must begin to explore the idea of donating their daughter's organs to benefit a number of other people. From the point of view of the uncomfortable health professional in this case, it is easier simply not to ask.

This issue of consent raises the following ethical questions:

- Does society have a right to the organs of an individual who dies in such a way as to be suitable for donation?
- Do all involved health professionals have a responsibility to ask for donation in every suitable instance?
- Is it unethical for an involved health professional to fail to ask for consent? Has he/she done the right thing for the grieving family? For those awaiting transplantation?
- Is it ethical to place the responsibility for a waiting recipient's imminent death on the family of a potential donor? Is this coercion?
- Is it morally acceptable for those health professionals who are involved in the care of transplant recipients to approach families for consent to donation or is this a conflict of interest?

A number of jurisdictions in North America have responded to these concerns by enacting legislation which places some of these issues under the aegis of the law. For example, required request laws stipulate that families must be asked for consent unless there is any other overriding contraindication. Consequences of failure to ask include non-payment of government insurance benefits to the institutions in some cases. However, even these laws do not provide complete answers to ethical questions posed about rights and responsibilities, as well as coercive approaches to obtaining consent.

Paid Donors

Another possibility for increasing the number of available organs for transplant is to commercialize the process and provide payment to donor families. Despite the fact that commercial trade in organs is illegal in North America, the possibilities of this approach continue to attract some people. If we do offer to pay donor families for organs, the following questions need to be answered:

- How much is a part of a human body worth?
- How would the exchange of money change the relationship of the donor to the caregiver? Of the recipient to the caregiver?
- Should we allow consenting adults to purchase live donor organs (i.e. kidneys) from consenting recipients? Should health professionals have any say in this private transaction?

As a consequence of the International Transplantation Society's stance against the practice of buying and selling human organs for transplant, discussion of these questions may be academic. At the present time, organ sale is not allowed in our society as it is in other countries such as India, where classified advertisements for the sale of kidneys and corneas by the poor appear in newspapers every day. But part of our problem in dealing with the new technologies is that we fail to anticipate future developments—which only too soon become everyday occurrences.

Living Donors

Until the past few years, the idea of using unrelated live donors for transplantation of solid organs was not an issue: it simply was not done in North American transplantation centers. But, the lack of cadaveric organs for transplant, coupled with successful new procedures, has made this a viable option. Living, unrelated donors are now used for kidney transplantation, but the procedure is usually restricted to what has been termed "emotionally related donors," which refers to spouses, close friends, step-relatives, etc. The ethical issues raised by these donations are decided on the basis of risks vs. benefits. There are potential medical and emotional risks and benefits to both the donor and the recipient, although the medical risks to the donor far outweigh any medical benefits. These need to be weighed carefully in any discussion of the use of living donors. Consider the following questions:

- Why is it considered appropriate to remove an organ for transplant from a consenting adult when that person is emotionally related to the recipient, but not otherwise?
- Do health professionals have the right to refuse to transplant an organ that is being offered by a competent adult, even if the recipient is not "emotionally related" to the donor?

- Do health professionals have the right to subject healthy individuals to the known risks of major surgery for organ donation even though they have expressed their willingness?

There are two sides to this dilemma, and the outcomes are never entirely happy regardless of whether we decide that it is or is not appropriate to look to unrelated live donors to increase the pool of available organs. First, we need to uphold the autonomy of an adult who chooses to make the altruistic act of giving an organ. On the other hand, we need to be assured that, along with this "good" that we seem to be doing (to the recipient), we do no harm (to the donor).

Anencephalic Donors

Another possibility that has been explored over the past few years, especially with the purpose of increasing the availability of organs for babies and small children, is the use of anencephalic infants. Born without an upper brain, these unfortunate babies have no chance for survival. However, they usually have normal hearts and other organs, and it seemed possible that they might make ideal donors for those babies awaiting heart transplant. As this procedure is becoming increasingly successful with babies in a number of centers, such as the well-known Loma Linda Medical Center in California, the need for organs will continue to grow.

However, many questions are raised about the use of these infants. In particular discussion has centered around the following issues:

- Are these infants "human" at all?
- Are these infants "alive" in any real sense?
- Can death be declared since the requirements for the declaration of brain death are not usually fulfilled in these cases?
- Should pregnant women known to be carrying anencephalic babies (which can be diagnosed prenatally on ultrasound) be encouraged to carry the pregnancies to term for organ donation?
- Is it appropriate for doctors, nurses, and technicians in intensive care nurseries, and more importantly parents, to be subjected to the stress involved in caring for these little creatures while death is awaited?

In North America at the present time, any such discussion is purely theoretical. Many moratoria have been placed on the use of organs from these babies until some of these questions can be answered adequately.

Use of Fetal Tissue

The transplantation of fetal tissue is another issue that fires the imaginations of the public and continues to spark fierce debates. Connected as it is with the abortion debate, the emotions generated by the notion of using fetal tissue for transplant all but completely cloud the real ethical problems that have yet to be addressed. Currently, fetal tissue is mainly used on an experimental basis for patients with Alzheimer's disease. Fetal tissue also has potential use in the treatment of Parkinson's disease and diabetes mellitus.

Some of the questions that need to be answered include the following:

- Is it ever ethical to view a pregnancy from a utilitarian perspective and allow a woman, for either personal or financial reasons, to become pregnant for the sole purpose of providing tissue for transplant?
- Is consent required from the producer (the mother) of the tissue for use of that tissue that would be otherwise disposed of, as in the case of a therapeutic abortion?
- Is it ethical not to use aborted tissue for its possible benefits when it will be destroyed anyway?

When an abortion will take place regardless of whether the tissue is used for transplant, not to use the tissue can be seen as tragically wasteful, not unlike the situation of a young person who dies and whose family is unable or unwilling to donate the organs. Perhaps, in this case, the donation of aborted tissue might assist the woman to deal with the sequelae of her decision to abort. The real problem, however, may lie in the future; if this practice becomes common, it is possible that the uterus might one day be considered an organ farm. The ethical knots need to be studied and untied before we can move on.

The Effects of Media Participation

The final issue in the discussion of donor problems is not the specific donor source, but rather one approach used to obtain organs. Without a doubt, transplantation is the medical field of most interest to the media, and two specific ethical issues arise from their coverage of organ donation.

First, transplant and organ procurement agencies throughout North America rely very heavily on the media, as well as their public relations efforts, to bring their message of the need for organ donors to the public. As a result, this field, that ought to be no more awe-inspiring than gastroenterology or proctology, has been glamorized. As high-profile programs bring more money into university teaching centers, conflicts can develop over allocation of limited funds. More money may be granted to transplantation than to other less publicized programs, because transplantation raises an institution's profile. Media attention can cloud the objectivity of even the toughest administrator or clinical practitioner.

The second, and probably more important ethical problem, results from the media appeals launched by desperate families who are searching for an organ for a loved one. This kind of publicity has both good and bad effects. Certainly, the attention of the public is drawn to the need for organs for transplant. However, that attention is almost completely centered on one individual patient and his or her plight. This may have the effect of disrupting the system of assigning available organs to the patient who needs it the most, not the one whose family's efforts have attracted the public eye.

A classic case of media intervention in the donation of an organ for transplantation occurred in the spring of 1986 when notification of a heart donor for Baby Jesse took place on national television on *The Phil Donahue Show*. The baby's parents, ages 26 and 17, were appearing as guests on the show after their baby had been turned down for a heart transplant by the team at Loma Linda Medical Center in California. They contended that one of the reasons for the refusal was that they were not married. When a donor became available and the announcement was made on television, public sympathy was focused on Baby Jesse, who was ultimately transplanted. According to an unidentified medical spokesman, had the usual computer search been done for a recipient after that donor had been found, it would have selected another infant awaiting a heart transplant, and that infant might well have been a more suitable recipient. Obviously, allowing organs to be donated with apparent name tags attached to them risks upsetting the precarious balance of objectivity that caregivers try to maintain in these difficult situations. Thus, media intervention is of concern because it may affect the selection of recipients.

Recipient Problems: Who Gets the Organs?

The ethical issues involved in the selection of recipients for transplant fall almost exclusively within the context of the ethical principle of justice. The allocation of human organs for transplant is part of the broader question of allocation of scarce resources in health care delivery. In this specific case, there are two questions to be answered.

- How can fair decisions be made regarding who should be transplanted in general and in each situation in particular?
- What criteria should be used to exclude individuals from transplantation?

Greatest Need Principle

In general, the candidates who are most in need of transplants and who have the greatest likelihood of having a successful outcome are the individuals who should and do receive the available organs. Problems arise, however, when, after using all of the strictly medical and objective measures currently available, no clear candidate emerges. This problem is probably best illustrated by the following response to American liver transplant surgeon Thomas Starzl's suggestion that the only thing the ailing 33-year-old Mozart needed to save his life was a kidney:

As appealing as such a historical mercy mission might be, there would remain the difficulty of finding a kidney for Mozart and then of deciding whether Mozart is more entitled to it than, say, a peasant, a charwoman, or, for that matter Salieri. (Lyon, 1987, pp. 46–47)

Exclusion Principle

As health professionals we must ensure that beneficial treatment is not withheld, but when the resource required is in short supply, we cannot offer treatment to everyone. One way of reducing demand is to exclude certain individuals from being considered for transplantation, despite the fact that transplantation might help them.

Who should be excluded from consideration for transplantation? For example, should we provide liver transplants for those individuals who have developed liver failure as a result of alcohol consumption? Should we deny smokers access to heart transplantation? Do we have the right to deny an illicit drug user a kidney transplant? Are these unwarranted value judgments on our part, or would exclusion of these individuals ensure that we are doing the greatest good for the greatest number?

As we have discussed previously, one of the pressing ethical dilemmas presented by the new technologies is that we are forced to look critically at the potential benefits and burdens of these procedures not only for individuals, but for future patients, and for society in general. Clearly, transplanting a liver into an alcoholic who has no intention of drying out or a heart into an individual who refuses to quit smoking would be viewed by other patients as unfair, because ability and willingness to comply with the medical regimen ought to be appraised when the medical criteria are considered. Moreover, society, in general, is likely to view allowing such people access to these procedures as excessively wasteful. While we cannot deny individuals the right to choose any lifestyle, neither does society have a responsibility to provide them with more than their share of health care services. The delivery of these services is premised upon the concept that each of us has some responsibility to maintain our own health.

Some transplant centers themselves are formally wrestling with this dilemma. In early 1990, the Ethics Committee at the University Hospital in London, Ontario, Canada's premiere transplantation center, issued a guideline to doctors saying that "patients who are willing to follow doctors' orders should get preference for a transplant over those who are not" ("Alcoholics get low priority," 1990). The Canadian Medical Association stated that this was the first time a hospital had issued a written guideline governing the allocation of this $110,000 liver transplant operation, which, in Canada, is an insured service under the provincial medical services insurance plans.

In addition, we need to consider the cost of these procedures in relation to other health and social services to which North Americans demand access. As University of Chicago psychiatrist Chase Kimball says, "You can feed a lot of hungry children on what it costs to do one heart transplant" (Lyon, 1987, p. 43). Another author asks:

> Is it appropriate for a relatively small number of people to benefit from public financing of an expensive technology when a larger number of people could benefit from expenditures on a broader range of less expensive health problems? (Kutner, 1987, p. 23)

Kutner (1987) draws several conclusions about the issues related to the costs of high-tech medical procedures and at least one of them is worth considering further. She suggests that "medical institutions know that transplant center status brings prestige, financial rewards, and the ability to expand related institutional programs such as immunology research" (p. 32). If used as a basis for the development and promotion of such programs, this consideration is in opposition to the application of any known ethical principles. In fact, the channeling of health care funds to further the ends mentioned above could be judged by society to be misappropriation of funds and, as such, unethical behavior.

Summary

This discussion of ethical issues in transplantation has merely scratched the surface of some of the problems in the specialty, most of which are related to scarcity of resources and a high media profile. As one prominent transplant physician has said, "Not that we are not moral or ethical, it is simply that within the very restricted confines in which we carry out experiments, the macro-ethics—the eventual implications of what we do—are not necessarily felt or understood" (Rauchman and Tan, 1987, p. 8). All of our individual actions added together may have major impacts on future directions.

Questions for Discussion and/or Review

1. How do you think that adequate numbers of organs can be secured for transplantation? Which methods would you advocate and which ones would you ban?

2. Discuss the legal and ethical problems of obtaining consent to secure organs.

3. On the whole, do you approve or disapprove of attempts to secure organs for specific patients through the media? Why or why not?

4. Should any restraints be placed upon media coverage and appeals? Who should define these?

5. How should the health system allocate organs for transplantation?

6. Are there any grounds, apart from scarcity, on which you think patients should be denied access to organ transplantation procedures?

7. What is the law where you reside concerning: (a) abortion, (b) use of fetal tissue, (c) organ donation, (d) recipient selection?

8. Discuss the ethical problems surrounding the use of organs from anencephalic babies.

Recommended Reading

Annas, G.J. "The Prostitute, the Playboy, and the Poet: Rationing Schemes for Organ Transplantation," *American Journal of Public Health*, 75 (February, 1985), 187–189.

Gero, Elaine and James Giordano. "Ethical Considerations in Fetal Tissue Transplantation," *Journal of Neuroscience Nursing*, 22 (February, 1990), 9–12.

Houlihan, P.J. *Life Without End: The Transplant Story*. Toronto: NC Press, 1988.

Parks, W., R. Barber and G.A. Painvin. "Ethical Issues in Transplantation," *Surgical Clinics of North America*, 66 (June, 1986), 633–639.

12

Medical Research: Experimenting on Humans

In this chapter:

- Examples of research on humans
- Estimating risks to subjects
- Obtaining consent
- Avoiding coercion
- Maintaining confidentiality
- Use of placebos
- Enticement of health professionals

There are in fact two things, science and opinion; the former begets knowledge, the latter ignorance.

Hippocrates

Science frees us in many ways...from bodily terror which the savage feels. But she replaces that, in the minds of many, by a moral terror which is far more overwhelming.

Charles Kingsley, 1866

An Historical Perspective

In 1796, Edward Jenner inoculated a healthy eight-year-old boy with smallpox and discovered vaccination. If he had been confronted with the ethical quagmire that we are about to present, it is quite possible that this discovery would have been significantly delayed. In fact, if Jenner and many of the other early medical researchers had been subject to the rigorous standards that are currently favored by those concerned with research involving human subjects, it is conceivable that some discoveries might never have been made. Indeed, *was* it ethical for Edward Jenner to subject a healthy young boy to the unknown risks of an untried medical approach? Or, on the other hand, does his success and the success of others indicate that the current concern about experimentation on humans is only modern hysteria?

As we have discussed previously, health care ethics is based on current morality and, although there are certain moral principles that would seem to be able to stand the test of time, health care research, like other issues in medical technology, must be considered in the context of the times within which it was or is conducted. With the increasing emphasis on the rights of the individual in recent times, ethical concepts in medical research have also had to evolve. "In the face of an evolution of ethical values and the recognition of cases of abuse, public policy has developed ethical codes to protect subjects of research" (Medical Research Council of Canada, 1986, p. 5).

In 1964 (revised in 1975), the World Medical Association adopted "The Declaration of Helsinki," a document which set forth guidelines for maintaining ethical standards in the implementation of medical research involving human subjects. However, the adoption of a code alone cannot solve problems, as illustrated by a number of situations in the United States, where the American Medical Association had adopted the Helsinki Declaration as its guideline for conduct of research.

One classic illustration of disregard for these principles came to be known as the *Tuskegee Syphilis Study*. Begun as a prospective study by the American Public Health Service in 1932, the study was designed to examine the natural course of untreated syphilis in 400 adult black males. In spite of the widespread availability of penicillin by the 1950s, the study carried on unimpeded until 1972, fully eight years after the adoption of the Helsinki Declaration, when public outcry finally made its continuation impossible. When the *New York Times*, *Time* magazine and others published details of the study in 1972, it seemed almost impossible that such actions could have been committed by those supposedly dedicated to doing good.

Unfortunately, abuse of human rights in the cause of advancing medicine has not been as uncommon as we might like to believe. We are all familiar with the atrocities carried out by Nazi medical experimenters in the name of science, which led to the adoption of the Nuremburg Code. More recently, in the 1960s and 1970s, situations closer to home involving abuse of human rights became public. For example, in the Hamburg State Home and Hospital, Berks County, Pennsylvania, researchers injected retarded children with a meningitis vaccine that had not been approved by the Federal Drug Administration in order to test its efficacy. Evidently, the researchers believed that approval of the hospital administrator constituted consent of a legal guardian and that this was sufficient (Foster and Raehl, 1980).

Health Care Research Today

Research is an essential part of the scientific basis of medicine today. Moreover, the more research done on human subjects, the more likely a diagnosis or treatment is to be safe and efficacious. Problems arise, however, when human beings are used as subjects in studies where the risks and benefits of treatment are unknown.

Criticism has been leveled recently against the medical profession for using treatment modalities that have little basis in scientific research. Rachlis and Kushner (1989) make three observations:

- Since most medical therapies have never been evaluated against rigorous scientific standards, there are significant unknowns in many treatment modalities.
- In medical school, budding physicians are exposed to the outcomes of scientific inquiry, but are not provided with adequate tools to analyze critically the basis on which conclusions are reached.
- As a consequence of the variability of quality in medical research, coupled with the fact that many physicians rely on published accounts of that research to update their knowledge, continuing medical education also lacks scientific rigor. (For example, for years doctors recommended and carried out tonsillectomies and adenoidectomies by the thousands, and allied health professionals continued to provide care for these patients, without any hard scientific evidence to indicate their usefulness. The number of children whose tonsils are whipped out has dramatically decreased as more medical

practitioners have begun to realize that the previous indications lacked scientific support.)

To a significant extent, the three observations above could easily be made about
any number of health professions. An inquisitive student nurse, upon inquiring
about the basis of particular approaches to patient care, from treatment of decubitus
ulcers to site selection for intramuscular injections, may still receive as an answer:
"Because that's the way we've always done it"—the ultimate in unscientific justification!

Health care research, whether initiated by pharmacologists, nurses, doctors, technologists, or even social workers and psychologists, involves many different
caregivers. Thus, in today's increasingly technological health care delivery system,
it is more important than ever before that each of us is cognizant of the requirements
for ethical research involving patients. While there is a need for clinical data, there
is also a need for each of us to play a role in protection of the health, well-being,
and human rights of the research subjects.

Areas of Ethical Conflict

Many of the ethical conflicts that arise in human experimentation are not unique
to this area of study. The following topics are, however, of particular concern in the
use of humans in health care experimentation:

- estimating risk to subjects;
- consent and coercion;
- confidentiality;
- placebo ethics;
- enticement of health professionals.

Risk vs. Benefit

A major problem in medical research is the inability to estimate, in a very precise
way, the risk to subjects of the treatment under investigation. In fact, if all risks
were known, the treatment would probably not be considered experimental. Thus,
estimating risk to subjects is the first issue for discussion.

The risk to a subject in a medical experiment can be placed on a continuum from
a situation of "no risk" (e.g. a patient receiving a placebo) on the one end to "life
threatening risk" (e.g. a patient receiving an artificial heart) on the other (Kopelman,
1981). The difficulty in using such a continuum in practice is the almost impossible
task of determining the precise amount of risk involved. One way of thinking about
the magnitude of the risk might be to use a simple decision-making framework
where all possible outcomes are evaluated for their magnitude, multiplied by the

Risk Assessment in Human Experimentation

	Magnitude	Probability	Risk
Outcome 1	X	=	
Outcome 2	X	=	
Outcome 3	X	=	

probability of their occurrence. The resulting risk of each outcome can then be measured. Figure 12.1 illustrates this operation.

The same operation can then be conducted to examine the benefits that may be accrued by the subject. The potential magnitude is multiplied by the probability of a beneficial outcome, and this product may then be subtracted from the total risk to get a broader picture of the risk/benefit ratio. Obviously, this process works better on paper than it does in practice, but it does provide a framework for determining the seriousness of risk, a procedure which is essential in order to ensure that the principles of doing good and doing no harm are followed.

If estimating risk is the first step in the ethical treatment of research subjects, then allowing the individual an informed decision and obtaining consent is the second. Herbert (1977) suggests the following rule for acquiring new information while maintaining old ethical standards:

> A person should not be subjected to avoidable risk of death or physical harm unless he freely and intelligently consents. (p. 693)

Consent vs. Coercion

The issue of the subject's consent vs. coercion to participate is another of the important ethical issues in health care research. Obviously, consent was not an issue for either Edward Jenner or the Public Health Service researchers in the *Tuskegee Syphilis Study*. Nor was it a concern for countless other medical researchers throughout history who lived in times when the concept of individual human rights was all but non-existent. However, the maintenance of patient autonomy is an important principle for the modern researcher. One of the ways that we do this is by providing the opportunity for and encouraging patients to have input into their health care decisions, especially those that involve the use of unproven procedures and pharmaceuticals. The important questions are: how much information can we provide to the patient and how is this best accomplished so that a truly educated decision can be made? These questions are of even more concern in the area of experimental procedures, with all its unknowns. The principle of allowing the patient to make an informed decision about whether or not to participate in a research study is essentially the same as that of obtaining patient consent to procedures under normal circumstances of health care. Patients, the prospective subjects, must be given enough information at a level they can understand so that truly informed decision making can take place, the obvious problems of dealing with children and incompetent persons notwithstanding. Basically, in order to make an informed decision a potential research subject needs information about:

- the kinds of risks and their respective probabilities;
- the magnitude and duration of each risk;
- the magnitude and probability of potential benefits;
- the safeguards for minimization of risk and maximization of benefit.

In the role of researcher, we must also keep in mind that the potential risks and benefits will not necessarily be the same for each potential subject; individual circumstances must be carefully considered. Thus, a standard consent form to be used for all subjects may be insufficient.

Patient coercion, in contrast to patient consent, is more of a problem in research than anywhere else in health care. Care must be taken to ensure that the patient is in no way made to believe that he/she *must* consent to be in the study in order to receive care.

One problematic situation may occur when the enthusiasm of the researcher subtly manipulates the patient into making a decision that might not be made if the facts were presented in a more objective way. The researcher's need for information might be construed to be in conflict with the patient's right to autonomy. Perhaps one way to obviate this possibility is to ensure that the principal investigator is not the person charged with obtaining the consent.

Patient desperation poses yet another problem. For those individuals suffering from terminal or otherwise extremely serious illnesses, the very idea of being helped may, on its own, be construed to be a form of coercion. For example, patients with AIDS are often willing to go to great lengths in order to obtain experimental drugs.

Further coercion of patients to participate in research studies and clinical trials may occur when a reward of some sort is offered for participation. Inducement may come in the form of money, free products, or an offer of free services; these constitute enticement. For example, drug companies occasionally recruit patients by offering the drug free at the end of the study period. Poor patients are particularly vulnerable to this kind of enticement.

As difficult as these issues are when dealing with a population of patients as potential research subjects, they are no less so, and may be even more of a problem, when students and/or other health care workers themselves might be suitable subjects for a study. In fact, the possibility that participation or non-participation in a study may affect an individual's career can comprise undue pressure and thus not allow the person to make a free consent. For example, a health professional student who is doing poorly in a particular professor's course might be tempted to become a research subject in hopes of boosting a flagging grade.

Maintenance of Confidentiality

The ultimate goal of any research exercise is to be able to predict, with a relatively high degree of certainty, the outcomes of an experimental treatment for larger populations than simply the study group selected. The degree to which the results of individual research studies can be generalized depends on several factors, including sample selection procedures, study design features, and statistical analyses. For any of the information gleaned from a study to be useful to other health professionals, the results must be communicated in some way. The publication of research results brings us to another ethical conflict in health care research, that of confidentiality.

Consideration of the right to privacy of an individual subject is the cornerstone of maintenance of confidentiality in health care research. Potential subjects have a right to be informed at the time they consent to participation about the dissemination of results. They need to know:

- how they will be identified, if at all;
- where and how the results are likely to be made public.

Safeguards of subject privacy must be built in right from the beginning of the study for the benefit of both the participant and the researcher. Voluntary participation in survey research, for example, can be significantly decreased if the subjects are not sufficiently comfortable with the explanations of how confidentiality will be maintained. In fact, in research that entails self-description of attitudes and/or behavior, a fear of identification can result in false data being collected, to the detriment of the study.

Use of Placebos

There are probably few other areas of research outside the health fields where placebos play such a significant role. Thus, a brief discussion of *placebo ethics* is warranted.

Dorland (1965) defines a placebo as "an inactive substance or preparation, formerly given to please or gratify a patient, now also used in controlled studies to determine the efficacy of medicinal substances." Quite apart from their controversial psychosomatic use in treatment in general, it is this latter use of placebos in clinical trials that concerns us here.

As a consequence of the deceptive nature of a placebo, there is an ethical risk of undermining the patient's autonomy, as well as the trust that the patient has in the caregiver. This, however, can be minimized by ensuring that, after disclosure of the potential risks and benefits, as well as the nature of the treatment selection process, the patient is given full control over consent to participate. In other words, the patient enters the study knowing that there is a possibility of being randomized into the group receiving a placebo, and its risks and benefits have been identified. Serious ethical problems are thus eliminated.

Enticement of Health Professionals

The final area of concern we have identified as important to the ethics of research is that of *enticement of health professionals* by organizations, primarily pharmaceutical companies, in the name of science. The best example is the post-clinical trial, the testing of drugs after they have already been approved for use. The sales representative for a drug company walks into a physician's office with a beautiful leather briefcase which he opens to reveal a supply of a particular medication, patient brochures, and a set of questionnaires to be completed. The physician is requested to participate in a post-clinical trial of the drug by placing six patients on it and filling in the questionnaires. At the completion of the study period, the briefcase becomes the property of the doctor. This scenario has been repeated countless times, and the "enticement" offered has ranged from trips abroad to personal computers. The ethical issue here is: are these trials truly contributing to the advancement of pharmaceutical research or are they simply creative marketing techniques?

Surely, if these trials were essential components of scientific inquiry, rewards for participation would not be necessary. In fact, caregivers should be more than eager to participate in the acquisition of new knowledge as a part of a well-designed research study, without gifts being given. The marketing representatives of these companies know that if the drug is reputable and efficacious, the physician prescribing it is unlikely to change the patient's prescription after the completion of the trial, thus increasing sales of the drug. The ethical problem presented here is the invasion into the relationship with the patient who trusts the physician to make treatment decisions based on his/her best medical knowledge without outside influence. The best way to handle this situation is to agree to participate, but to refuse the gift. Thus, agreement to participate is based on what is believed to be best for the patient, no outside influence has been exerted, and perhaps a contribution to science is

Standard Values and Obligations in Health Care Research

VALUES	OBLIGATIONS
1. To do good	1. Risk assessment
2. To do no harm	2. Disclosure
3. To maintain patient autonomy and confidentiality	3. Informed decision making

Figure 12.2.

actually being made. If the physician cannot see his/her way clear to participate under these circumstances, then he/she ought to refuse.

We present these issues not as an exhaustive discourse on health care research, but as a starting point for thought and discussion on the ethical component of scientific inquiry. Careful consideration of these questions can provide a basic framework for assessment of ethical research participation.

Summary

It is essential that the researcher be aware of and demonstrate certain philosophical values and moral obligations to ensure that health care research is conducted in an ethical manner. Figure 12.2 above summarizes these standard values and obligations.

Maintenance of the basic principles of doing good, doing no harm, and respect for patient autonomy and confidentiality require the researcher to assess the risks, make full disclosure at a level that the subject can understand, and provide opportunity for an informed decision. In addition, the researcher should ensure that no undue pressure is placed on either the potential subject or the researcher him/herself.

Scientific inquiry is one of the few ways that health care delivery can be validated. Even if we are not engaged in the process as researchers ourselves, it is the responsibility of all caregivers to ensure the ethical conduct of studies in which they or their patients participate.

Questions for Discussion and/or Review

1. What precautions should be taken before any medical research on humans is carried out? What patient rights need to be considered?

2. What are the policies in your workplace regarding such research?

3. How can confidentiality of results be maintained?

4. What safeguards should the physician maintain in protecting patients in the use of new drugs?

Recommended Reading

Carico, Janice and Elaine Harrison. "Ethical Considerations for Nurses in Biomedical Research," *Journal of Neuroscience Nursing*, 22 (June, 1990), 160–163.

Connolly, T.J. "Willing Participant or Exploited Patient?" *Medical Journal of Australia*, 1 (February 21, 1981), 172–174.

Kopelman, Loretta. "Estimating Risk in Human Research," *Clinical Research*, 29 (February, 1981), 1–8.

Smith, Harmon. "Ethical Considerations in Research Involving Human Subjects," *Social Science and Medicine*, 14A (1980), 453–458.

13

AIDS and Ethics

In this chapter:

- The scope of the problem

- The fundamental dilemma: The rights of the individual versus the rights of society

Diseases desperate grown
By desperate appliance are relieved,
Or not at all.

William Shakespeare, *Hamlet*, Act IV, Scene iii

At present AIDS is a contagious and incurable disease. It arouses strong emotions, challenges our deepest values, and has a very high media profile. All these factors combine to make this particular disease the source of ethical dilemmas that appear more unyielding with each passing day.

In the not so distant past, before antibiotics and vaccinations, caregivers commonly faced the possibility of contracting tuberculosis, smallpox, diphtheria, typhoid, cholera, and polio. But today, the infectious plague of AIDS is being treated by health professionals who rarely have been required to face that kind of personal risk. Today's caregivers have also been educated in times when antibiotics are regarded as a golden bullet. They are generally unused to caring for people, often young, with a specific disease who are as yet beyond help.

Over the past decade, the problem of HIV infection and what to do about it has forced a whole generation of health professionals in every discipline to confront more ethical health care problems than have ever been raised before. It has served to arouse an intense interest in ethics and ethical issues in the general public as well. For this, if for nothing else, we can be grateful.

The Magnitude of the Problem

It might seem odd that a textbook on health care ethics should devote an entire chapter to the issues related to one particular disease, a disease that, to put it in perspective, currently affects a relatively small number of people on this continent. In fact, in absolute terms, the morbidity and mortality associated with heart disease and cancer far outweigh the rates associated with HIV infections, as this is written. Why, then, does this disease warrant such an in-depth discussion?

Before 1982, few health professionals had even heard of anything resembling AIDS. At that time, the disease process had only recently been dubbed acquired immunodeficiency syndrome, a change from its former name, Gay-Related Immune Deficiency (GRID). Originally thought to be confined to the population of homosexual men, the disease was now known to be transmitted by blood transfusions, and intravenous drug users were identified as another population at risk. It was only a matter of time before other at-risk populations were identified. By 1983, the newly named human immune virus itself had been isolated in the blood of affected patients, and researchers began to communicate their findings to a wider audience.

If the number of papers in the literature is an indication of the magnitude of concern expressed by health professionals, then AIDS and the issues that surround it are perceived as an ever-increasing problem. In a study of the medical literature between 1983 and 1987, 412 papers were examined. While the general references to AIDS and HIV increased by about one-third annually, the number of papers related to ethics and AIDS doubled with each year (Manuel et al., 1990). Clearly, AIDS is a very serious disease, and the recognition of the ethical problems it creates is growing rapidly.

There are two medical aspects of this disease which make it of particular concern from an ethical point of view. First, in North America, at present, AIDS is an infectious condition wherein the mode of transmission is, to a significant extent, related to lifestyle choices. This factor thus raises issues of homosexuality, multiple sexual partners, use of prophylaxis for sexually transmitted diseases, and intravenous drug use, all of which are value-laden. Second, as far as is known at present, AIDS is always fatal; it cannot yet be cured by modern medicine. The terminal nature of the condition creates far more serious ethical dilemmas that are, in modern times, inherent in the processes of dying and death. In addition, issues related to allocation of resources are raised, because the care required to deal with these usually young patients to their untimely deaths is intensive and expensive. These considerations have not been seen in combination during the lifetimes of the vast majority of health professionals working today. Thus, concern about the personal risk of contracting a disease which is infectious, incurable, and fatal is a very real problem in dealing with infected patients. Many of today's caregivers are young themselves, and the victims of AIDS are often their age or younger. In no other illness is the health professional's fear of death so acutely challenged as in situations where he/she must watch helplessly as the victims succumb.

A study carried out by a behavioral scientist and reported in the mass media discovered that medical students have what was described as an exaggerated fear of contracting AIDS ("Medical Students Fear AIDS...," 1990). The survey of 548 medical students also found that their general attitudes indicated prejudice against people who have the disease, with half of them expressing the opinion that medical students should have the right to refuse to treat HIV-infected patients.

The Fundamental Dilemma: Conflicts of Rights

The fundamental dilemma posed by the so-called AIDS epidemic can be summed up simply: conflicts of rights—rights of the patient versus rights of the caregiver and of society. There are several such conflicts:

- the individual patient's right to privacy vs. the right of significant others (e.g. contacts) to know;

- the individual patient's right to privacy vs. society's (including the caregiver's) right to be protected;
- the right of the individual to needed treatment vs. the rights of others for access to scarce health care resources;
- the individual's right to receive care vs. the health professional's right to refuse treatment.

Three Obligations to Patients

Generally, when dealing with ethical dilemmas, we need to work from a series of presumptions which may be overridden if sufficient justification exists. We often use the basic principles of ethical conduct to guide us; in the case of the health professional dealing with the AIDS dilemma, we need first to be clear about our primary obligations to the patient. We are committed to:

- give the best care that we can;
- be honest;
- be trustworthy.

As simple as these obligations may seem, keeping them firmly in mind helps put into perspective the decisions that we may have to make in extraordinary circumstances, such as those presented by the AIDS issue. How, then, can we fulfil our obligations to the patient while, at the same time, seeking a solution to the conflict of rights?

The Obligation to Treat Patients

First, to give the best care that we can does not imply that health professionals necessarily have the obligation to treat everyone. In fact, those patients who, for one reason or another, you may feel that you cannot provide care for would probably be better served by someone else. The obligation to provide unquestioning care, as set out by the various codes of ethics, is usually only required in emergency situations. However, it is clear that this interpretation of our obligation would run into difficulty if every caregiver refused to treat a certain type of patient, in this case, HIV-infected patients. The reason for refusing to treat these patients does not stem from a moral objection (as might exist in the case of abortion, where refusal has been considered justifiable). Instead, the avoidance of these patients in most cases may be directly attributed to the caregiver's fear of contracting the disease. What, then, can be considered a reasonable level of risk to which health professionals must be willing to be exposed?

By definition, individuals who choose careers in the helping professions are exposed to significantly more health hazards than those who choose not to become health professionals. There are built-in risks to the health occupations that must be accepted. Thus, to name but a few, the family physician who is exposed to numerous communicable diseases on a daily basis, the radiotherapy technician who is continually exposed to minute doses of radiation, and the nurse who risks back injury by moving a heavy patient all face hazards. Grady (1989) reviewed the literature to determine the relative risk of contracting AIDS and concluded that the risk is too small to warrant refusing to treat these patients. (Although a small risk does exist, the likelihood of contracting hepatitis B is 20 to 30 times higher.) One medical association discussion paper (Gilmore and Somerville, 1989) indicates that "unreasonable refusals to care for patients with HIV/AIDS are ethically unacceptable…" (p. 30).

Another controversial aspect of our obligation to provide the best care that we can relates to the allocation of scarce resources to patients infected with this terminal disease. As the numbers of infected patients continue to grow, the cost of the intense care required to care for them until they die becomes astronomical. The absolute futility of all that we are currently able to do also adds weight to the argument that the care given to these patients should be rationed. Patients with HIV, however, have the right to be cared for, with their needs being compared with the needs of patients with other illnesses, and the resources being used accordingly. However, resources should currently be targeted at halting the spread of the disease in order to eliminate the need for increasing treatment services in the future.

The Obligation to Be Honest

The second primary obligation to the patient is to be honest. This implies upholding the patient's right to know about his/her condition and the treatment alternatives, and to play a part in the decision-making process. It also implies that we must be honest and forthright in dealing with conflicting rights. For example, you need to make known to the patient your legal obligation to report sexually transmitted diseases to the authorities. You must also advise the patient of any personal biases that may prevent you from fulfilling your first obligation—to give the best care that you can. Turning the tables, however, poses even more perplexing questions. How honest does the HIV-infected caregiver need to be with the patient?

In a nationwide survey of 2000 Americans, researchers at the University of California at San Francisco found that 45% of respondents believed that physicians who are infected with HIV should not be allowed to continue to practice (Gerbert, Maguire, Hulley and Coates, 1989). Surely, then, if the caregiver has the right to know which patients pose a risk, albeit small, to them (a belief that does not enjoy a consensus with either health professionals or patients), then patients must have the right to know the HIV status of all caregivers, although the risk of the patient contracting the virus from a caregiver is estimated to be even smaller (Dickey, 1989). It would seem to work both ways, but, in fact, it probably works neither way.

A past chairperson of the American Medical Association's Council on Ethical and Judicial Affairs has indicated that physicians, and by extension other caregivers, should be allowed the simple civil liberties that are afforded to other citizens, namely, "the right to privacy and the right to work so long as others are not at risk" (Dickey, 1989, p. 2002). Since she postulates that no real documented risk to the patient exists, then there is no obligation for the caregiver to provide information on his/her own HIV status to the patient. The argument over the definition of "risk" in the case of AIDS and health care workers continues in the literature, and each year will bring changes in that definition.

In early 1991, media reports of a Florida dentist who apparently infected a number of his patients with HIV sent shock waves through the dental community, as well as the general public. According to the reports, he wore gloves and a mask, strategies which are supposed to protect both caregivers and patients. Following this perplexing discovery, the American Dental Association recommended to its members that AIDS-infected dentists tell their patients of their condition or stop performing invasive procedures. The Canadian Dental Association continues to regard this as an isolated case and has not made recommendations to this effect (Taylor and Mickelburgh, 1991). Dentists are simply given the recommendation to inform their provincial licensing board if they are infected, but it is suggested to them that they do not inform their patients.

The Obligation to Be Trustworthy

The third basic obligation that we have to patients is to be trustworthy, with the implied responsibility not to reveal that which needs to be kept confidential. As we have discussed previously, the belief that health professionals will respect confidences is one of the factors that encourages patients to disclose all relevant information to the benefit of treatment. It is, however, difficult to keep to the letter of this obligation when failure to breach that confidence may potentially harm others. Many health professionals believe that the importance we place on patient confidentiality in the case of AIDS is misplaced and that our obligations to society far outweigh any obligations to the individual patient. However, since society's perceptions about AIDS can result in considerable negative social and even financial consequences for the patient, the decision to disclose a person's HIV status cannot be taken lightly. In addition, we need to be aware that wholesale breach of confidentiality may prevent some individuals who may be infected from seeking testing and may thus contribute to the spread of the disease. At the very least, being trustworthy means that caregivers have the responsibility to inform the patient if confidences must be shared with other specified individuals.

The delineation of our three basic obligations cannot answer all the questions that are posed by the AIDS problem, but they serve as a framework for discussion of our own values and beliefs and how these can be rationalized with long-held principles. Caregivers need to be aware that any answers to these questions may not indicate the views of the majority. There are almost as many perspectives as there are health professionals.

The Desperate Patient

As Shakespeare says in the introductory quotation to this chapter, desperate diseases have spawned desperate cures or none at all. This has never been more true than in the case of AIDS. With modern medical technology as yet unable to cope with this deadly malady, patients searching for a reprieve, if not a cure, have been forced to look to a variety of unconventional sources for help.

When there is no proven treatment available for a fatal disease, any news of discoveries, no matter how small, raises the hopes of the victims, often to unrealistic heights. On two occasions in 1985, announcements of "breakthroughs" in France were made, and many desperate Americans headed to Paris in the hope of finding the miracle cure. Blame for the subsequent dashed hopes has been placed both on the researchers for releasing the information without adequate scientific foundation and on the media for inflating the stories out of proportion. Regardless of who was at fault, these situations illustrate the problems encountered in dealing with desperate patients. Should patients with terminal diseases have access to novel therapies that have not yet received the legally required testing and approval?

There is, of course, a conflict here. First, the individual's right to autonomy in decision making must be upheld; but, as health professionals, we also have an obligation to protect patients from quack remedies. One recommendation for dealing with this problem is to:

> ...assist a patient with HIV/AIDS to obtain a novel therapy on a compassionate basis, when the patient expressly requests...it, unless...the risks and harms...outweigh the benefits and potential benefits...(Gilmore and Somerville, 1989, 32)

Caregivers should be available to assist the patient to make an informed decision and to support whatever decision follows.

Summary

AIDS is a serious medical, social, economic, and ethical problem, perhaps, indeed, the most serious situation ever faced by health professionals. This disease has already created a significant number of very contentious dilemmas and will undoubtedly continue to do so for some time to come. Caregivers need to consider carefully their own value systems as they struggle with the dilemmas created by this disease and apply the principles that guide the ethical decision-making process.

Questions for Discussion and/or Reading

1. Does a health professional ever have the right to refuse to treat a patient? If so, under what circumstances and why? If not, why not?

2. When a patient has AIDS, whose rights take precedence—those of the individual patient involved or those of society? State the principles that support your opinion.

3. Do you agree with mandatory testing for the HIV virus? Discuss your reasons for supporting or rejecting the practice.

4. Does a caregiver with AIDS have an obligation to reveal this to patients? To other professionals? Why or why not?

5. What level of health care support do you think AIDS victims are entitled to? Should all medications be paid for, even experimental ones? Should hospice care be available to all?

Recommended Reading

Berger, Philip. "AIDS and Ethics: An Analytic Framework," *Canadian Family Physician*, 34 (August, 1988), 1787–1791.

Chiodo, G.T. and S.W. Tolle. "Doctor-Patient Confidentiality and the Potentially HIV Positive Patient," *Journal of the American Dental Association*, 119 (November, 1989), 652–654.

Cornblatt, M.S., M.J. Ayres and E.L. Kolodner. "A Legal Perspective on AIDS," *American Journal of Occupational Therapy*, 44 (March 1990), 244–246.

Grady, Christine. "Ethical Issues in Providing Nursing Care to Human Immunodeficiency Virus-Infected Populations," *Nursing Clinics of North America*, 24 (June, 1989), 523–533.

Hansen, R. "The Ethics of Caring for Patients With HIV or AIDS," *American Journal of Occupational Therapy*, 44 (March, 1990), 239–242.

Kerr, C.P. "AIDS and the Issue of Confidentiality," *Postgraduate Medicine*, 81 (June, 1987), 95, 98, 101.

Manolakis, M.L., G.M. McCart and R.M. Veatch. "Pharmacist's Refusal to Serve Patient With AIDS," *American Journal of Hospital Pharmacy*, 47 (January, 1990), 151–154.

14

Issues in Death and Dying

In this chapter:

- The high-tech death

- Euthanasia

- Rehumanizing death

- Living wills

- Costs of dying

Rage, rage against the dying of the light.

Dylan Thomas, 1952

Death is only a horizon.

Carly Simon, 1990

We must now turn our attention to the ethical dilemmas that occur at the end of life, just as we examined those at its beginning. Depending upon your point of view, death is either to be prepared for and accepted as inevitable, or is to be feared and loathed, even struggled against. Judging from the efforts of modern health care to keep us alive, medical technology and its proponents appear to regard death with all the horror one usually reserves for an enemy in war.

The end of human life now involves many moral problems which are directly related to the advances of high-tech medicine and its awesome capability for pro-longing "biologic" life. Just a century ago, death was regarded as a part of the normal cycle of life in most homes, where the actual dying process often took place. In the 1990s, most deaths occur in the sterile environs of the modern hospital, surrounded by the arsenal of modern medicine waiting for a chance to snatch the dying person from death's jaws yet one more time, and thus, too often, the dying process is simply prolonged. With this frightening and exhilarating power to play God so easily available to health professionals, there is often an overwhelming temptation to forget that part of our responsibility is to assist the patient in the accomplishment of a peaceful death.

Some current problems in this area involve making difficult decisions about when modern medicine should withdraw and allow the normal human cycle of life and death to take over. As our technology sustains the lives of the seriously ill, the ethical implications of removing treatment must be examined. We need to examine our own values about death and dying, not just as caregivers, but also as human beings, in an effort to put humanity back into an increasingly technology-driven event.

The High-Tech Death

North American society has, over the past century, become steeped in a bone-chilling fear of death. We have fought against this inevitable end to life with every weapon of medical technology, and the result has been to increase dramatically the average life expectancy. While most of us welcome the longer and healthier lives that have been a major legacy of medical research, this success also raises the question of when we should stop, both in general terms and in individual situations.

Every health professional working in hospitals has witnessed countless scenes of what has come to be known as the high-tech death. In this event, instead of a nurse or a doctor sitting quietly with the family, holding the patient's hand and easing him or her into a peaceful death, as soon as the patient breathes for what would have been the last time and the flat line appears on the cardiac monitor, the medical wheels start spinning. Crash carts are rushed into the room; residents, interns, respiratory therapists, nurses rush to the scene. A cardiac board is slid under the patient's back, and as the endotracheal tube is slipped expertly into the trachea, someone kneels up on the bed, takes charge of the heart, and begins the chant, "A thousand and one, a thousand and two, a thousand and three…" The person in charge of the lungs begins the inflations and synchronizes them with the cardiac compressions. The person in charge of the blood chemistry readies syringes, while others take notes and charge up the defibrillator. Compressions, inflations, defibrillations, injections begin and are continued in succession until either the patient's heart reluctantly says, "Enough, already," and wearily begins to beat again, or the team becomes too exhausted to continue. The old person's eyes flutter open, look around at the white-coated bodies, and with considerable confusion, he or she asks, "Am I dead?"

The question anyone new to this scenario is bound to ask is: "Isn't anyone allowed to die anymore?" No longer is the technique of cardiopulmonary resuscitation restricted to its original purpose—to treat individuals in emergency situations when the expected outcome was a long life—but is commonly used for dying patients who just happen to be in the hospital (Buckman and Senn, 1989). CPR is one of the most basic of weapons in the technological arsenal and is a good starting point for discussions of the fundamental moral questions that surround the modern concept of death. These include:

- When should people be allowed to die?
- Who should decide when a person should be allowed to die?
- How should the decisions about death be made?
- What measures should be permitted in allowing the individual patient to die?

Death vs. Cardiac Arrest

In recent years, many health professionals have fallen into the trap of considering CPR as a treatment for every death that occurs in the hospital. In other words, they fail to differentiate between the 45-year-old woman in the final stages of metastatic breast cancer, the 45-year-old man who has just suffered a myocardial infarct, the 80-year-old woman with Alzheimer's disease, or the six-year-old child suffering from profound hypothermia. In effect, by treating all these patients as though they would all benefit from CPR, they obviate the necessity of facing the ethical dilemmas raised by the following questions:

- Does CPR do any good for the patient?

- Does CPR protect the patient from any harm?
- Is this what the patient would want?

Buckman and Senn (1989) suggest several criteria that can assist us to identify those individual patients who clearly should not be subjected to cardiopulmonary resuscitation. Patients who would not benefit from the procedure and who meet the following criteria would *not* be considered candidates for CPR:

- those who suffer from an irreversible and fatal condition;
- those whose current treatment is palliative only;
- when death is expected within a short time;
- when the above criteria are verified by an independent physician.

Such criteria provide us with a starting point for individualizing our approach to treating the death of a patient and for developing a consensus within the health care system for application of procedures such as CPR.

Nurses, in particular, face difficult situations every day of their professional lives. As the caregivers who spend the greatest number of hours with a patient, they are most likely to discover the patient who has suffered cardio-respiratory death. Without clear, well-established, and agreed upon criteria, such as those presented above, the nurse is in the unenviable position of having to decide either not to call a code or to summon the cardiac arrest team, regardless of what is in the patient's best interests. We need to consider these interests both from our point of view as caregivers, as well as from the point of view of the patient.

Giving Death a Helping Hand: Euthanasia

Euthanasia, commonly referred to as mercy killing, is more and more widely and frequently the subject of discussion in both the popular press and the professional literature. Based on the belief that individuals have the right to decide when their lives should be terminated, euthanasia has attracted more interest recently for several reasons. People are becoming more and more resistant to the attempts of the medical profession to prolong life at any cost. As the concept of patient autonomy has become more acceptable to the health professions, demands are growing from the general public for less medical interference in the process of dying. The traditional arguments about the sanctity of life are now being countered with pleas to consider what quality that life contains. In recent years this idea has gained in acceptance. A considerable number of celebrated cases have brought the issue into the forefront of medical ethics discussions, as moral decisions about a time to die have been eclipsed by legal ones.

One of the most publicized cases of this nature involved a 26-year-old, mentally competent quadriplegic woman in California who chose to end her life, pitting her individual rights against the obligations of the health professionals. A patient in a hospital at the time, and physically unable to end her own life, the young woman asked that the hospital provide her with hygienic care and painkilling drugs and allow her to starve to death. When the case reached the superior court, the judge acknowledged her right to end her own life but ruled that the hospital staff could not be compelled to stand by and watch her die. Accordingly, intravenous feedings were begun.

The specific ethical implications of giving death a helping hand should be considered within the broad context of several of our basic general ethical principles, namely, to do good, to do no harm, and to uphold the patient's right to self-determination. We also need to keep in mind that, although advances in medical technology have given rise to new questions regarding when death ought to be helped along, the concept and discussions about euthanasia are as old as civilization, dating back to the Greeks and Romans.

Daniel Callahan provides us with a perspective on the need to renew discussions on euthanasia:

> The power of medicine to extend life under poor circumstances is now widely and increasingly feared. The combined power of a quasi-religious tradition of respect for individual life and a secular tradition of relentless medical progress, creates a bias toward aggressive, often unremitting treatment that appears unstoppable. (Callahan, 1989, p. 4)

What is the difference between homicide and euthanasia? When the principle of sanctity of life is interpreted in its most literal and extreme sense, there is no difference between the two. In fact, the current laws in North America seem to support this position. If, however, human life is held to be more than simply a vegetative state, there is considerable difference, whether you find the concept of euthanasia supportable or not. The difference between murder and euthanasia is one of consent: murder is committed against the will of the victim; euthanasia is carried out at the wishes of the patient. Conceptually, then, killing and euthanasia are two different things. This differentiation, however, does not necessarily place one in the realm of the ethically moral and the other, the ethically immoral. Further examination is necessary.

The next difference to define is the difference between active and passive euthanasia. Many caregivers are becoming fairly comfortable with the concept of either withholding or withdrawing treatment that is clearly not having a beneficial effect on the patient, even if this might hasten the individual's death. In other words, they accept the concept of passive euthanasia *under certain circumstances*. However, active euthanasia—carrying out procedures known to hasten a patient's death—is a concept that is more difficult for health professionals to come to terms with.

Caregivers must accept public input into future decisions on the morality and legality of euthanasia. In fact, if we, as health professionals, bury our heads in the sand and fail to come to grips with this issue, it will inevitably be decided for us by some other authority. Then we may find ourselves in the position of having to act on the basis of policies and laws that we find insupportable, based on our own personal value systems, as well as because of our professional opinions of what is best for the patient.

One thing is clear at present: public opinion polls on euthanasia have been consistently in favor of the practice. In a 1986 Gallup poll in California, 70% of respondents answered affirmatively when asked: "Should adults who are terminally ill be allowed to legally end their lives?" (Parachini, 1989). In the Netherlands, euthanasia under specified circumstances is already considered a medical, not a legal matter. However, on this continent, the American Medical Association has taken the consistent position of opposing the practice.

In a recently reported American study (Kuznar, 1991), almost 10% of the physicians who responded indicated that they had deliberately taken action to end the life of a terminally ill patient, with over 90% reporting that they had given a do-not-resuscitate order. Less than 4%, however, had ever given a dying patient information about committing suicide. Considering the popularity of the 1991 book *Final Exit: the Practicalities of Self-Deliverance and Assisted Suicide for the Dying* by Derek Humphrey, the issue is of increasing concern to the general public.

In late 1991, the voters of Washington state had an opportunity to voice their opinions on the right-to-die issue as they participated in a referendum on a bill that would make their state the first political jurisdiction in the western world to legalize euthanasia. However, the voters did not support the passage of the bill, indicating the difficulty of coming to a clear position on this issue.

Moral positions both in favor of and in opposition to euthanasia can be equally convincing. If we have a right to life, then we ought also to have the right to death; as caregivers, we may have the responsibility to assist in that death and thus uphold the patient's right to self-determination. On the other hand, support for euthanasia can be viewed as the slippery slope down which we may slide toward the elimination of those individuals in society who are viewed as unproductive—the sick, the deformed, the elderly—and, indeed, may represent to some the antithesis of why most of us entered the helping professions in the first place. Whether, in your view, euthanasia will benefit or harm the patient depends upon how you view death, but the determination of benefits and burdens ought to be made by the patient, assuming that the patient is competent to make this decision. (We will discuss the issue of incompetence later.)

Active and passive euthanasia cannot be either morally or legally acceptable, however, unless a basic trust exists in the relationship between the caregiver and the patient. The patient must have sufficient trust in the caregiver to believe that euthanasia would be practised only at the request of the patient, not on the basis of a paternalistic decision by the caretaker that it was in the patient's best interests. The important question for the North American health care delivery system is: do patients trust us enough?

Rehumanizing Death

How to resolve the fundamental question of the relative importance of quality of life as opposed to quantity of life lies at the heart of the dilemmas surrounding the dehumanizing of the dying process.

In a celebrated case in 1990, the parents of a 32-year-old woman, Nancy Cruzan, asked the US Supreme Court for permission to end their daughter's life. This was not a case of a decision to turn off life support systems after a patient had suffered brain death. The parents' request was based on the argument that quantity was not the yardstick to measure life for this unfortunate young woman, who had lain comatose in her hospital bed since 1983, when a car accident had rendered her severely brain damaged. The decision of the Supreme Court indicated that she could be allowed to die if there was *clear and convincing evidence that she would want to*. Although she had not left such written instructions, a former co-worker testified that the patient had stated she would never want to live this way, and the petition to disconnect her feeding tube was granted.

Clearly, this legal decision provides civil protection for American health professionals who might come to the ethical conclusion that, in the interests of patient dignity and autonomy, measures should not be taken to prolong life. And from a moral point of view, it is certainly arguable that if patients have left specific instructions about their wishes under these circumstances, then those wishes ought to be given the highest priority. One of the ways that we can be assured of our position in individual situations is to encourage the use of living wills.

Living Wills

Every day, in medical offices and hospitals across the continent, health professionals are engaged in taking the medical history of their patients. A new concept, the "medical future," is now becoming just as important as this history, perhaps more so because of technology (Kapp, 1988). Among other things, a medical future includes descriptions of the patient's wishes about future health care in an effort to uphold his/her autonomy and prevent unnecessary indignity, suffering, and pain at the hands of an overzealous caregiver. These documents have been called a number of different things, most commonly, living wills and advance directives, but their purpose is the same—to allow individuals to maintain the right to self-determination in situations where they are no longer able to voice their own wishes (see Appendices).

Living will legislation was first enacted in the US in California in 1976, and similar laws have since been passed in most other states (Greaves, 1989). In addition, as of November 1, 1991, all health-related organizations serving Medicare or Medicaid patients must provide any new adult patient with written information about his/her legal rights as a patient, including the right to a living will. This "Patient Self-Determination Act" provides powerful encouragement for the use of advance directives (Singer, 1991). Several Canadian provinces, including Nova Scotia and Quebec (others are pending), have also enacted living will legislation. Simply having laws on the books, however, does not ensure that they will be followed. In fact, since the enactment of the first laws, their actual usefulness in practice has been limited by restrictive interpretations on the part of health care personnel, as well as by the parameters of the laws themselves. For example, some of the legislation is so worded that it can only be applied when the patient is terminally ill. In the case of Nancy Cruzan, for example, although she was certainly not living a life as most of us know it, she was not, in fact, terminally ill in even the broadest interpretation of the term. Thus, although these laws do provide a certain amount of protection for the professional integrity of the caregiver, as well as the self-determination of the patient, their usefulness is limited. The fundamental premises upon which decisions regarding living wills are made must obviously be moral, not legal.

As caregivers, we need to become comfortable with the idea that when a person is ready to die, we need not necessarily jump to the rescue and destroy the dignity of the process. There are those who take the idea of sanctity of life so seriously that they believe that only God has the right to make the decision to end life. However, we know that it is not God, but high-technology health care that often prolongs the dying process.

The High Cost of Dying

When people talk about the high cost of dying, they are usually referring to the seemingly inflated costs associated with caskets, funeral homes, and memorial services. They seldom consider the costs associated with the events leading up to the need for these services. In fact, many caregivers, as well as others, think that there is something inherently inhumane about discussing how expensive it is to care for an individual throughout the process of dying. With escalating health care costs, however, it is only prudent that in consideration of the greater good, we give some thought to just how much these prolonged lives are costing us.

According to Dr. Frederick Lowy, Director of the Centre for Bioethics at the University of Toronto, Canada's publicly-funded health care system could potentially save four billion dollars if elderly patients were given the option of refusing unwanted life-extending care (Rich, 1990). He based his computations on US 1990 estimates that of the total $661 billion to be spent on health care, almost 30% ($184 billion) would be spent on 6% of the population—those elderly patients covered by Medicare who would die during that year. Further, Lowy estimated that about $150 million would be spent for life-extending treatments that the patients may not even have wanted, since only 10%–15% would be capable of discussing these matters with their physicians.

The "life of any type, at any cost" philosophy of some health professionals is clearly inappropriate given rising concern for the greater good. We are not alone in our belief that:

> ...the relation between the economic and moral dimensions of care for the terminally ill is a subject that can be addressed openly, without embracing a crude calculus that trades life for dollars. (Bayer et al., 1983, p. 1490)

We are not suggesting that, because we cannot rationally expect a favorable "return" on our expenditures in caring for the dying patient, we should cease to make the investment. What we are saying is that reasonable decisions about how to be cost-conscious can be made without dehumanizing the care of the dying. Bayer and others (1983) have suggested three goals for development of cost-containment policies. These include the need to:

- develop clear criteria for admission to critical care units;
- promote patient and family autonomy;
- promote alternative forms of institutional care, such as hospices.

Objectives of this nature can provide us with both a starting point for discussions to clarify our own values in this area and a method to rationalize the decisions that will surely have to be made in future.

Summary

We would do well to consider this thought from an article entitled "A Time to Die," originally published in *The Economist*:

> Think of a person's life in biographical rather than biological terms—in terms of achievements, experiences, responsibilities discharged...not in terms of blips on a hospital scanner. It then becomes easier to see when somebody's life has been completed. When a person (or his relatives)

can see that a biography is finished, it is not for doctors to try to write a painful extra chapter. ("A Time to Die," 1990, p. 986)

Questions for Discussion and/or Review

1. Give examples of patients for whom CPR is an appropriate procedure and for whom it is not.

2. Do you think euthanasia is morally acceptable or unacceptable? If so, on what grounds?

3. Define the difference between active and passive euthanasia and state whether or not and why you support either, both, or none.

4. How do you think the health care system can best help the dying patient?

5. Does your workplace have a policy regarding living wills? If so, state what that position is. If not, state what you think the position should be.

Recommended Reading

Crump, William J. "Helping Your Patient Prepare a Living Will," *Senior Patient*, (March–April, 1989), 85–86, 91–92.

Gibbs, Nancy. "Live and Let Die," *Time*, (March 19, 1990), 52, 54–58.

Miller, Phillip J. "Death With Dignity and the Right to Die: Sometimes Doctors Have a Duty to Hasten Death," *Journal of Medical Ethics*, 13 (June, 1987), 81–85.

Various authors. "Mercy, Murder and Morality," *Hastings Center Report*, special supplement, 19 (January–February, 1989).

Part III

The Practice

15

Good Manners:
Etiquette and Ethics

In this chapter:

- ■ Why manners matter

- ■ How and why relationships within the profession are changing

- ■ Components of professional good manners

- ■ Practical problems of professional conduct

    - Whistle-blowing

    - Strikes and/or work stoppages

    - Sexual relationships with patients

Independence? That's middle-class blasphemy. We are all dependent on one another, every soul of us on earth.

George Bernard Shaw, *Pygmalion*, 1912

Evil communications corrupt good manners.

I Corinthians, 15: 33

The concept of good manners is usually given short shrift in most discussions of ethics. However, our professional conduct does and will play a vital part in decision making in all areas of health care. If the advances in health care of next century are anything like those of the present, then we, as health professionals, need to look to our colleagues in our own disciplines, as well as to those in other allied health groups, for consultation and support. We will need each other's help in dealing not only with the technological innovations, but also with the moral questions. Respect for one another, then, will be the cornerstone of our interprofessional relationships. In addition, plain, simple, human respect for our patients, demonstrated by good manners, may be one of the few ways in which we will be able to sustain mutual trust in the face of increasing consumer skepticism. Good patient care is only possible in an environment that sustains that respect, even in situations of question-able jurisdiction between caregivers of varying backgrounds. We are not Emily Post, but we believe that professional etiquette provides a personal framework for dealing with the thorny ethical problems presented by modern health care.

The Renaissance of Good Manners

Ethics and etiquette are similar in that both attempt to provide guidelines about right and wrong behavior. One definition of etiquette—"rules conventionally established for behavior in polite society or official and professional life,"—could, if the words "polite society" are removed, almost pass for a definition of ethics. Currently, there is a revival of interest in etiquette and good manners. One has only to browse through the business section of a bookstore to see a plethora of guides on business etiquette, providing advice on everything from what to eat at a business luncheon to whether or not one ought to sleep with colleagues or clients. On the other hand, guides to etiquette in professions outside the business world are not as easy to find. And we do need some guidance in making a variety of decisions in situations unique to modern health care delivery.

For example, how do you deal with:

- the power struggles between members of different disciplines;
- the questions of overlapping jurisdictions—the "turf" problems;
- the changing roles and educational status of some of the health disciplines;

- when you should "blow the whistle" on an incompetent colleague or a colleague with a problem that could possibly affect competency;
- the decision to participate in a strike;
- the question of whether you should ever become involved in a non-professional relationship with a colleague? A patient?

These are some of the practical questions of behavior that are not addressed in discussions of current ethical issues, but that comprise many of the day-to-day concerns of the caregiver. Some will be discussed in more detail later in this chapter.

There is no one discipline that makes the modern health care delivery system in North America function; a variety of professionals and non-professionals alike are required to provide optimum care for the patients. Doctors cannot provide health care without nurses; nurses cannot provide care without doctors or technicians. We each have a specialized role to play. Before we begin to examine some of the finer points of professional etiquette that sustain this system, we need to consider the basics of simply getting along together.

Elena Jankowic, a business etiquette consultant, defines the "Golden Rule of Business" as *everyone is important* (Jankowic, 1986). We need to keep this in mind as we learn to operate in the health professions. Basic respect for everyone involved in health care, from the chiefs of staff and the administrators down to the laundry workers and porters who deliver the trays of food, smooths our working relationships. It also allows us to consider other points of view. When mutual respect underlies the daily working relationship, it is natural, faced with difficult problems, to solicit and consider input from a variety of disciplines to the ultimate benefit of the patients.

Relationships Past and Future

The traditional hierarchical relationships among members of different disciplines in the health professions are no longer as clear or as rigid as they once were. No longer is the doctor necessarily considered to be on top, with everyone else merely acquiescing to his [*sic*] every whim. This shift in attitude has been caused by three major societal trends: a change in the roles of women, the scientific explosion, and the education explosion.

The Effects of Feminism

The shift in women's traditional roles from work inside to outside the home has changed the faces of both the medical profession and the nursing profession, the largest single health discipline. Approximately half of all the new medical students today in North America are women; this dramatic increase is beginning to affect the power base of the profession. In addition, women in the nursing profession, which is still approximately 97% female, are no longer content with the traditional rules of the game. According to Stein, Watts, and Lowell (1990), "the cardinal rule of the game was that open disagreement between the players had to be avoided." In 1967, when one of these authors examined the game and described it in the literature for other physicians, "nurses needed to communicate their recommendations without appearing to make them. Physicians requesting a recommendation needed to do so without appearing to be asking for it" (p. 546). Today's nurse, physiotherapist, occupational therapist, or speech pathologist is more likely to give an opinion or recommendation and expect that it will be followed or, at the very least, considered, in the medical treatment of the patient.

Not all physicians, however, are happy about how this is playing itself out. A young female physician writing a letter to the *New England Journal of Medicine,* in response to the analysis by Stein, Watts, and Howell tells it from her perspective:

> As a young female physician, perhaps I am more sensitive to this issue of hierarchy. Some nurses resent receiving orders from a younger colleague and offer resistance at every turn. I am tired of defending literally every order I write. Question me when it is warranted, show me my mistakes when I have made them, but give me some credit for my years of college, medical school and postgraduate residency training. Also, remember that in the eyes of the patient and my colleagues, I am ultimately responsible for your actions as well as my own. (Munday, 1990, p. 201)

In Jungian psychological terms, familiar archetypes and images underlie the traditional relationships. The physician can be seen to represent the father or god, and the nurse, the mother or handmaiden (Schattschneider, 1990). While these images in the subconscious minds of the patients may be comforting, they serve the traditional status quo, and do nothing to further our abilities to learn from each other. This is especially important in situations where the expression of differing perspectives is crucial to doing the right thing. Situations requiring ethical reasoning also demand the acceptance of a variety of viewpoints, despite the importance of personal values. Open and direct communication with our colleagues is the first step in the development of the respect that is so vital to the provision of excellent and compassionate patient care.

The Effects of the Scientific Explosion

As we have discussed previously, the scientific explosion has had an enormous impact on the practice and delivery of health care. The expansion of specialized knowledge, coupled with technological advance, has resulted in the development of the many and varied health care disciplines we know today, each with its own area of expertise. Not all of the boundaries of the "turfs" are agreed upon though. For example, within the two disciplines with the longest histories, doctors claim to have been usurped by nurses, and nurses claim to have been usurped by everyone from practical nurses to health educators. As we come to know, understand, and respect each other's areas of expertise, we will be able to spend less time on jurisdictional disputes and more time on patient care.

The Effects of the Educational Explosion

Finally, the educational explosion has added yet another facet to interprofessional relationships. As competition for places in professional schools has heated up, requirements for admission have leaned even more toward academic excellence, arguably to the detriment of the personal characteristics and value systems which may be part of an ability to provide humane care. One has only to hear discussions between first-year medical students just after they have received their first-term marks to understand how important maintaining the competitive edge is to them.

However, with increasing frequency, we can read in the professional literature discussions of how to develop most effectively a compassionate caregiver. For example, some medical schools are looking critically at their use of the Medical College Admission Tests as a major criterion for admittance. Some argue that the preparation required for successful performance on these tests tends to slant the pre-medical education further and further away from the humanities and more toward the pure sciences. Medical educators are becoming less sure that the doctor resulting from that course of study possesses the characteristics ideal for physicians.

A further concern is competition between the professions. For example, changes in the required levels of education for some caregivers have left their colleagues in the other disciplines disturbed. The movement in North America toward a requirement for a baccalaureate degree as the entry level to the nursing profession has resulted in confusion among others, such as physicians, who do not understand the objectives of these changes and may be uncomfortable at the thought of competing with nurses. It is still possible to read in the medical literature opinions which reveal dislike and disdain towards higher education in nursing and other allied health professions. It would seem far more worthwhile to try to understand how much more these professionals have to offer as a result of their higher education than to bemoan the perceived loss of unquestioning obedience.

While the development of new health care disciplines and higher levels of education have undoubtedly resulted in new methods of relating to colleagues, new behaviors have also emerged in old relationships, such as those between doctors and nurses. It is not helpful for us to look back and despair for the loss of the old ways, but instead to look forward to how we might best function within the new roles. Interprofessional dialogue is a necessity so that we may understand and respect each other, not seek to control.

The Components of Professional Good Manners

All health professionals should have a shared set of professional and personal values. These are the essence of professional good manners.

We present, for your consideration, our "Rules of Behavior for Health Professionals."

Focus on Your Own Work, Not on the Work of Others

If each caregiver were first concerned about doing an exemplary job within his/her own discipline in a manner congruent with a personal set of values, patients would be assured of better care. Undue attention on the work of others, such as the physician's often inordinate concern about what the nurse is doing, constrains the autonomy of the individuals and downgrades their disciplines, with unfortunate ramifications for everyone in the system.

Be Conscientious about Your Own Work

In order to be conscientious we must accept personal responsibility and be accountable. Honesty, reliability, and follow-through are also necessary to produce work that is above reproach. As we have already determined that your personal value system underlies your ability to contribute to ethically defensible decisions, this rule is a fundamental necessity in your professional life.

Be Cautious about Self-Disclosure

Consider the scenario of a physician who discloses details of his or her weekend activities to a patient in general conversation. When the doctor reveals a penchant for wine and cigarettes, credibility with this patient, and any others to whom this patient may talk, is seriously undermined. As a result, the doctor's attempt to persuade this patient, who is suffering from heart disease, that he ought to quit smoking and decrease his alcohol intake may be less successful.

This kind of indiscreet behavior can be equally destructive to professional relationships. For example, co-workers may assume that, because of some of the doctor's extracurricular activities, he or she may be less reliable in certain situations, such as surgery. While we recognize that a certain amount of self-disclosure is a part of the therapeutic relationship, each of us needs to exercise some thought and caution before we speak.

Give Credit where Credit Is Due

This holds true whether the credit is due a colleague in your own or another discipline. A professional does not take credit for the work or ideas of others. The doctor does not pretend that the nurse's suggestion of how the medical regime for the patient might be organized was originated by him or her, nor does the nurse take credit for the post-operative care plan constructed by the physiotherapist. An individual who persists in taking another's work or idea as his/her own is displaying a lack of self-confidence and is undermining the smooth working relationships that are so necessary in today's complex health care delivery systems.

Take Responsibility for Your Own Actions

Although assuming responsibility is part of being conscientious, it is such an important attribute that it needs to be noted separately. The surgeon who faces difficulty at the operating table and blames the scrub nurse for the way she/he handed him/her the suture disturbs both colleagues and the working environment. Blaming other people when things go wrong is inappropriate and irresponsible and contributes nothing to the betterment of patient care.

Subscribe to a Code of Conventional Politeness

It may seem absurd even to mention this; however, we have all seen breaches of ordinary good manners in professional situations. Ask yourself the following questions:

- Do you always say thank you to the person who assists you with procedures (even when it is part of that person's job to do so)?
- Do you always say thank you when someone goes out of his/her way to help you?
- Do you always say please?
- Do you never reprimand a person (whether a subordinate or not) in the presence of others?
- Do you always keep your temper in control? (Angry scenes often occur in operating rooms.)
- Is your language always appropriate?
- Do you never make sexist remarks? Ethnic slurs?
- Do you refer to others with the degree of formality that you expect for yourself? (For example, if you expect to be called "Dr. Doe," don't call all the nurses by their first names unless they have given their individual permission.)

If you can honestly answer yes to all of these questions, you are probably known for your graciousness and courtesy, two ingredients that are often in short supply in

---

Summary of
"Rules of Behavior for Health Professionals"

- Focus on your own work and not that of others.

- Be conscientious about your work.

- Be cautious about self-disclosure.

- Give credit where credit is due.

- Take responsibility for your own actions.

- Subscribe to a code of ordinary politeness.

Figure 15.1.

---

hospitals and health care offices. Patients can sense when their caregivers have respect for each other and feel assured that they, too, will be treated with dignity.

Good manners are not an anachronism in the 1990s; there is always time to be polite. Even the most brilliant surgeon who has made international contributions to the advancement of medical science is not exempt from the rules of good behavior for a health professional. We each have the right to expect polite consideration from our colleagues.

Conflicting Obligations

In this discussion of the elements of individual good behavior, we need to be clear that we have obligations to behave well in our relationships with patients, with society, and with each other. These obligations, however, do come into conflict from time to time; there are three areas, in particular, that bear examination.

"Whistle-Blowing"

The first issue of conflicting obligations concerns what is known as "whistle-blowing." The question of when to expose a colleague who is incompetent or unethical directly involves a conflict between our obligations to society and our obligations to support other professionals. The preamble of the American Medical Association's Principles of Medical Ethics states: "A physician shall...strive to expose those physicians deficient in character or competence, or who engage in fraud or deception." The code of the Canadian Medical Association has a similar dictum, which refers to reporting conduct that is considered "unbecoming" to the profession. The International Council of Nurses' Ethical Concepts applied to Nursing indicates that the nurse should take "appropriate action to safeguard the individual when his care is endangered by a co-worker..." Other codes contain similar guidelines.

The reality of exposing an incompetent colleague is much more daunting than it might appear from reading a code of ethics. You may find it difficult to "blow the whistle" for the following reasons:

- The individual in question may be your friend.
- You may believe that it is really none of your business.
- You may be able to rationalize his/her behavior to yourself.

And after taking the courageous step of doing something about a problem that you perceived, you may be met with distrust from your colleagues who may wonder whom you plan to expose next. However, keep one thing in mind. When done diligently and with respect, exposure upholds the dignity of the patient and of the profession. Remember also that the person doing the reporting is not ultimately responsible for the outcome for the individual involved. That is the responsibility of the disciplinary body of the profession.

Strikes/Work Stoppages

The second issue which involves conflicting obligations is the question of whether or not health professionals ought to take part in strikes or work stoppages of any nature.

Such actions are often defended as being undertaken, at least to some extent, on behalf of patients, i.e. to ensure better quality of care for patients in the future. When caregivers go on strike, many issues to be negotiated do relate both directly and indirectly to the future of patient care. For example, it is clear that low wages and poor working conditions are partially responsible for the exodus of nurses out of their profession. Therefore, care that might otherwise be provided if sufficient numbers of experienced nurses were hired may be compromised. The clout of unions through the use of the strike weapon is often seen as the only way to improve this situation.

However, whatever the rhetoric, strikes primarily serve the needs of the workers who choose to withdraw their services. Strikes and work stoppages are weapons to gain certain ends. We are not interested in engaging in a discussion of the fundamental worth of trade unions and what they have contributed to the work world of today; we are only interested in making sure that each health professional who walks out on patients, for whatever reason, has a clear idea of whose needs are being served.

In this situation, the individual caregiver's obligation to provide patient care comes into direct conflict with the obligations that he/she has toward the profession. It is the case, which must be faced by the individual professional, that patients do suffer during the stoppage and that the caregiver is choosing to ignore the obligation to provide care. This is not to say that strikes are wrong, only that it may not be as simple as it first appears to the young professional faced with this wrenching decision.

The Canadian Medical Association's 1987 document on interpretations of the code of ethics provides some guidelines by recommending that:

> ...the ethical physician who, because of the characteristics of his/her work is a member of a trade union or association with the independent right of strike action, will always place his/her obligation to patient care and support of the Code of Ethics above adherence to the rules of the trade union or association. (Canadian Medical Association, 1987)

Whenever health professionals go on strike, it is headline news; the media is filled with dramatic stories of patients who cannot receive needed care. Regardless of how morally defensible the work stoppage might be, it imprints negative images in the minds of the patients and the public who rely on health professionals for care. Strikes are weapons that ought not to be brandished carelessly.

Forbidden Sex

> *I will stand free from any voluntary criminal action or corrupt deed and the seduction of males or females, be they slaves or free.*
>
> Hippocratic Oath

Even in the days of Hippocrates, the issue of forbidden sex was raised. The phrase "sex in the forbidden zone" was coined recently by a Californian psychiatrist, Dr. Peter Rutter, in his book of the same name. He defines this as "any sexual contact that occurred within professional relationships of trust" (Rutter, 1989, p. 11). While his examination explores the dynamics of male-female power relationships, and he indicates that his premise refers specifically to men in helping professions and their involvement with female patients, the reverse can also be true. Caregivers who are women are also capable of these indiscretions.

The issue of power, which we examined in more detail when discussing our relationships with patients in general, is of particular concern when the potential for an intimate relationship surfaces. The protective nature of the caregiver's relationship with a patient is shattered when a sexual involvement develops, regardless of who initiated it. Because of the nature of our obligations to the patient and the essential inequality of our interactions, sexual relationships are *always* wrong. It is the clear responsibility of the caregiver to recognize when the potential for such an involvement exists and take action to avoid it.

Summary

What should be clear by now is that the pursuit of individual independence and dominance is rapidly giving way to an era where professional interdependence is paramount (Zilz, 1990). We need each other and can no longer afford to see other professionals as appendages to our own work. Good manners and respect are the cornerstones for good health care relationships.

Questions for Discussion and/or Review

1. Why are professional manners so important? Give as many reasons as you can for maintaining polite conduct in your work.

2. Give specific examples from your own working experience of each of the components of good manners outlined in this chapter.

3. Discuss a working situation in which good manners played a part. How did they contribute? Describe a situation in which bad manners were displayed. How did this affect the people involved and their work?

4. What are the advantages and disadvantages of the traditional medical hierarchy?

5. Under what circumstances do you think it is essential to report a colleague's misconduct? Are there other situations and circumstances that you think do not require reporting?

6. Why is it generally agreed that sexual relationships with patients are *always* wrong? Do you agree?

Recommended Reading

Marsden, Celine. "Ethics of the Doctor-Nurse Game," *Heart-Lung*, 19 (July, 1990), 422–423.

Stein, L.I., D.T. Watts, and T. Howell. "The Doctor-Nurse Game Revisited," *New England Journal of Medicine*, 322 (February 22, 1990), 546–549.

Zilz, David A. "Interdependence in Pharmacy: Risks, Rewards and Responsibilities," *American Journal of Hospital Pharmacy*, 47 (August, 1990), 1759–1765.

16

The Ethicist and the Hospital Ethics Committee

In this chapter:

- ◼ Why we need ethicists and institutional ethics committees

- ◼ Functions of the ethics committee
  - Education
  - Policy development
  - Case consultation

- ◼ Composition of the ethics committee

- ◼ How caregivers interact with ethics committees

It is better to be a human being dissatisfied than a pig satisfied; better to be Socrates dissatisfied than a fool satisfied. And if the fool or the pig, are of a different opinion, it is because they only know their side of the question. The other party to the comparison knows both sides.

John Stuart Mill, *Utilitarianism*, 1863

When you know a thing, to hold that you know it; and when you do not know a thing, to allow that you do not know it—this is knowledge.

Confucius

The first step in decision making is always to identify the problem correctly. If, however, we fail to identify any problem at all, then, as far as we are concerned, no problem exists. Unfortunately, ethical problems in modern health care often remain unseen or are ignored. As health professionals, our heavy responsibilities for the clinical components of the care of the patient, which involve decisions about medical, diagnostic, nursing, and other regimes, often cloud our abilities to see any underlying ethical problems that may exist.

In 1981, when interest in a possible role for ethicists in health care delivery was beginning to emerge, a study of the inclusion of a physician-ethicist in ward rounds was reported in the medical literature. In the baseline or preliminary observations, the house staff and/or attending staff identified fewer than 4% of the patient cases as involving ethical problems. When a physician-ethicist attended the rounds, the identification of ethical problems rose to more than 15% of the cases (Lo and Schroeder, 1981).

The first step, then, in any solution to the ethical dilemmas of modern health care, is to improve our ability to recognize when a problem exists. As the study above indicates, we cannot assume that the majority of caregivers possess this skill. On the one hand, maybe we need help from a specialist. On the other hand, perhaps we may then see problems that are not really there.

Modern Health Care Meets Philosophy

The idea of consulting a specialist in health care ethics is another result of advances in modern medical technology. As the numbers of medical ethical dilemmas rose, so, too, did the need for people trained in the domain of moral reasoning, and, true to the trend toward increasing specialization, the medical ethicist emerged. Hospitals throughout North America began to seek out consultation and help in ethical matters, if for no other reason than to avoid costly legal battles. Over the past decade, caregivers have called upon philosophers, lawyers, and theologians to assist in the ethical decision-making process. The term "ethicist," however, is so new that it is not yet easy to find in a dictionary. A medical ethicist is a philosopher with expertise in ethical theory and a special interest in its applications to medically related issues and situations.

The purpose, then, of using the services of a medical ethicist is to obtain help in the identification and solution of ethical problems in health care delivery. As Professor Arthur Schafer notes, to use an ethicist is to hire a moral firefighter (Schafer, 1986). This is not to say that we ought to expect definitive answers from these consultants, only assistance in reaching those answers.

There are many people, however, who have suggested that this sort of consultation leads not to more answers, but to more questions. It is true that the very nature of the philosopher's approach to weighing conflicting values and subsequent arguments is likely to result in recognition and consideration of new dilemmas that the clinicians never suspected existed. After all, one of the main objectives of the study of ethics is consciousness-raising. However, the discovery of unsuspected problems can actually be of benefit, because we will be made aware of what we may have overlooked and thus avoid mistakes. In the fourth century B.C., Aristotle wrote that "the least initial deviation from the truth is multiplied later a thousandfold." In our attempt to find the truth, we may need a little initial help to prevent those later disasters.

Moral Consensus: The Ethics Committee Phenomenon and Its Functions

With the recognition of the need for interdependence in our practice and for assessing a number of viewpoints, the creation of the institutional ethics committee was inevitable. In 1976, a legal judgment recommended using such a committee to confirm the prognosis of a comatose young woman, Karen Ann Quinlan, prior to termination of her life support systems. After that beginning, ethics committees have evolved from providing support for medical decisions to moral decision making.

Ethics committees can have a number of functions, and differ from the research ethics committees that exist to evaluate the ethical soundness of research proposals involving human subjects in hospitals. We will examine three of their potential functions.

Education

First, the institutional ethics committee ought to have as one of its primary mandates the education of health professionals about modern dilemmas in health care delivery. Although ethical theories and ethical behaviour more commonly are being studied by students in health professional schools, the caregiver is rarely actually exposed to real ethical dilemmas in health care until he/she has graduated and entered the practice setting. Prior to this time, the degree of responsibility of the practitioner has been so limited that involvement in the identification and solution of ethical problems has been minimal. Upon graduation, everything changes. Suddenly, all those theoretical models that were used to explain ethical decision making and all those principles and guidelines that were learned take on an entirely different perspective. At this point, the ethics committee has a responsibility to continue the education of practitioners who may have forgotten those ideas that seemed less important than the scientific content of their various disciplines.

In addition, many caregivers working today graduated long before discussion of ethical problems became a common part of the basic educational preparation of practitioners. Despite their long experience in the delivery of health care, many of these individuals will require even more opportunities to discuss ethical concerns in the context of modern thought. The ethics committee can help these people to understand the current approaches to identifying and solving moral problems.

Policy Development

Second, the ethics committee ought to have input into institutional policy development. More and more health care organizations are now developing policies to assist them in dealing with recurring dilemmas, such as do-not-resuscitate orders, use of anencephalic newborns as organ donors, withdrawal of treatment in the terminally ill, and a host of other problems. Ethics committees become one of the most useful tools for developing recommendations on acceptable behavior for caregivers in these problematic situations. The committee can fulfil this function by taking on the role of researcher and analyst, examining both the theoretical basis of the problem and the empirical information available in the health care literature. In addition, the committee can seek documented public and legal opinion during the process of formulating policy recommendations. In this way, administrative strategies will be more effectively designed to reflect the moral tone of the society in which they must be implemented, and to provide a measure of protection for the caregivers who will put them into practice.

Case Consultation

Although considered by many to be the primary role of the institutional ethics committee, case consultation is probably the least important of the three roles. If the first and second functions, education and policy formulation, are fulfilled adequately, most ethical problems in health care delivery can be satisfactorily solved by those caregivers who are directly involved with the actual patient. There are, however, instances when the caregivers in question may be unable to come to a decision; they and the patient or family may then look to the institutional ethics committee for objective consultation.

Caregivers need to exercise some caution when consulting with ethics committees in individual patient cases. As some authors suggest, "The strongest argument against ethics committees engaging in case consultation is that it may interfere with the doctor-patient relationship and lead to worse, not better, care" (Fleetwood, Arnold, and Baron, 1989, p. 141). Thus, this argument assumes that a faceless, distant group of individuals who are not ultimately accountable for patient outcome can create a wedge between the patient and the individual caregiver. We need to strike a balance between using what has been referred to as the "moral authority of consensus" (Moreno, 1988), which we may consider to be inherently more objective, but which remains a concept by no means entirely clear, and maintaining the sanctity of the relationship between the patient and the individual caregiver. In fact, even the American Hospital Association's own guidelines state:

> Ethics committees should not serve as professional ethics review boards, as substitutes for legal or judicial review or as "decision makers" in biomedical ethical dilemmas. An ethics committee should not replace *the traditional loci of decision making on these issues* [emphasis ours]. (American Hospital Association, 1983)

Composition of the Ethics Committee

Now that we have discussed what roles the ethics committee might play, we need to consider who the members of this committee should be. The composition of any committee will have a direct bearing on the usefulness of its input into education, policy making, or case consultation.

There is considerable agreement that ethics committees ought to draw their members from both inside and outside the health professions. Typically, the health professionals sitting on ethics committees are mainly physicians and nurses. Given the current rate of technological advance in health care and the inclusion of ethics as a topic of discussion in a variety of allied health disciplines, we need to encourage broader representation from other groups. Technologists of various sorts ought to become valued members of these committees, as should therapists, psychologists, pharmacists, and others as deemed appropriate to the individual institution and situation.

Debate continues over the question of who the non-medical members on ethics committees ought to be. Members have been lawyers, administrators, clergy, ethicists, and social workers, all of whom have different perspectives to offer. In addition to these non-medical professionals, we strongly support the inclusion of lay people who will represent the community within which the health care organization provides service. As potential patients and family members of actual and potential patients of the institution, these individuals will, no doubt, provide another point of view that may be lost if only professionals with a job to do are included. Including community residents is a first step in addressing the on-going concern for public participation in making ethical decisions that may have long-term implications for health care delivery.

Obviously, anyone who becomes a member of an institutional ethics committee must be completely supportive of the aims and purposes of the committee and must be prepared to study and learn. Anyone who does not believe in the mandate will hamper the committee's work and should not be included.

Your Relationship to the Ethics Committee

Short of being a member of the ethics committee yourself (which is something you might consider), your relationship with the committee will, from time to time, likely involve the following roles:

- referring cases to the committee;
- taking part in educational seminars and discussions;
- suggesting issues that need to be explored in educational seminars and discussions;
- adhering to policies that have been developed based on the recommendations of the ethics committee;
- making a patient care decision based on a specific recommendation of the committee.

We will examine some of these situations in more detail.

Case Referral

Let us look at your role in the referral of individual patient cases. We have already suggested that this is not a procedure that should be followed every time a dilemma presents itself. In fact, remember that bringing in outside consultation is usually a last resort.

Who is the person who usually brings cases to the committee? Doctors, nurses, social workers, clergy, and other caregivers often identify a problem and bring it before a committee. As well, patients themselves, or their families, may also approach the committee for assistance in solving a problem. Individual hospital guidelines should be broad enough to allow such diversity in the origin of the consultation.

Education

When you take part in the educational opportunities offered by the ethics committee, you implicitly recognize an obligation to broaden your knowledge in the area of health care ethics on an on-going basis. Although moral principles do not change rapidly, their applications do. With each advance in the science of health care delivery, we are faced with new and confusing situations to which we must apply familiar guidelines. Taking part in educational programs and discussions allows us to consider many of the dilemmas long before we may encounter them. In fact, as you see developments in your own area of expertise, you might ask yourself: "What would happen if...," and thus discover new topics that you can suggest be explored in an educational program on ethics.

Following Recommendations

While you might use the recommendation of an ethics committee as the basis on which to make an ethical decision, such decisions are still ultimately the responsibility of the individual caregiver. Although you might seek the input of the group, until such time as that accountability changes, you are not obliged to follow its counsel. Be advised, though, that a good committee takes both moral and legal considerations into account when giving direction. So, if your own values lead you in a different direction, go in that direction cautiously.

Summary

It seems only fitting that in facing moral plurality and confusing ethical entanglements we should look to individuals or groups who might provide us with assistance in the formulation of sound moral decisions. Ethicists and ethics committees are here to stay, and their roles in the future need to continue to be monitored. The next step, of course, is the formulation of public policy to solve these thorny problems.

Questions for Discussion and/or Review

1. What roles can the ethics committee play? In what way do you think such committees can make the most valuable contribution?

2. When, if ever, do you think ethicists or ethics committees should be called into individual cases?

3. Who do you think should sit on the ethics committee?

4. What problems do you think might result from growing reliance on such committees?

5. What are the limitations of institutional ethics committees? Of medical ethicists?

Recommended Reading

Agich, G.J. and S.J. Youngner. "For experts only? Access to hospital ethics committees," *Hastings Center Report,* 21 (September–October, 1991), 17–24.

Fleetwood, J.E., R.M. Arnold and R.J. Baron. "Giving Answers or Raising Questions?: The Problematic Role of Institutional Ethics Committees," *Journal of Medical Ethics*, 15 (September, 1989), 137–142.

Levine, Carole. "Hospital Ethics Committees: Questions and Answers," *Hospital Trustee*, (November–December, 1986), 9–11.

Moreno, Jonathan D. "Ethics by Committee: The Moral Authority of Consensus," *Journal of Medicine and Philosophy*, 13 (November, 1988), 411–432.

17

The Sands of Moral Reasoning

In this chapter:

- ■ A process for ethical decision making
  - Collect information
  - Distinguish between needs and wants
  - Consult legal and ethical guidelines
  - Examine moral responsibilities
  - Uphold patient autonomy
  - Evaluate possible solutions
  - Make the decision
- ■ A word of caution

For the things we have to learn before we can do them, we learn by doing them.

Aristotle

Unlike philosophers, who have the luxury of time to spend considering many ethical theories when presented with a problem, and whose decisions usually have no immediate repercussions, the health professional must confront ethical dilemmas and make workable, practical decisions that have very real and immediate outcomes for very real people. The stock-in-trade of the philosopher is the discussion of different ways of thinking about issues and problems. Health professionals must act quickly, and accountability for decisions in health care still rests with them. Thus, in this book we have attempted to take a practical look at the issues facing the modern health professional, while avoiding abstract philosophical arguments that might cause the caregiver to give up and ignore ethical considerations when making decisions.

However, we have yet to discuss a model for how those decisions might be made. We have examined basic principles and modern issues and now we need to put them together to provide health care workers with guidelines to help them to apply the theories.

The Percolation Plan for Ethical Reasoning

Picture a cutaway view of the earth's crust. As rain pours upon the surface, water slowly begins to percolate through denser and denser layers of soil and rock whose composition becomes finer the more deeply we penetrate. As the water flows through these layers, perhaps small traces of minerals are left behind. Synthetic water purification works in the same way, and the final result is water that is free of the impurities it contained as it fell from the sky or was polluted by man. In the same way, we can examine ethical dilemmas in a systematic way that allows us to free them from contaminants as we progress toward a solution.

Thus, we are suggesting our percolation approach. Figure 17.1 illustrates, in diagrammatic form, how the "Sands of Moral Reasoning" provide us with the framework for using this percolation approach. Let us examine it step by step.

Collect Information

The first step in the process of ethical decision making is to gather as much appropriate and correct information as possible. Only when as many accurate details of the situation as we can find are before us can we identify the problem and search for appropriate and workable solutions. We need to answer the following questions:

The Percolation Approach to Ethical Decision Making

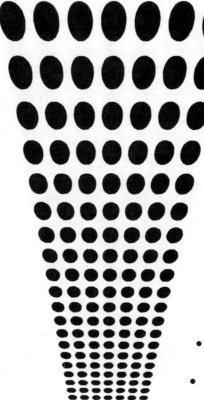

- Gather appropriate and correct information

- Differentiate between needs and wants

- Examine relevant civil laws and codes of ethics

- Consider your moral duties

- Ensure consideration of patient autonomy to the fullest extent possible

- Determine whether proposed solution represents benefit or burden and to whom

- What is my decision?

- Upon re-examination of my decision, do I need to filter any of its components and from what point?

Figure 17.1.

- Do I have all of the information?
- Is the information correct insofar as I am able to determine?
- Have I exhausted all available sources?
- Is there any hidden agenda among the pieces of information?
- Has my communication with others been adequate?

Differentiate between Needs and Wants

Once we are reasonably certain that we have all of the available information from all sources, we must distinguish needs from wants. Adler (1985) defines a need as a natural desire and a want as an acquired one. Our needs, therefore, are always good for us, while our wants may or may not be. We *ought* to desire a thing because we need it. However, this is not always the case. Our social priority is to meet the basic needs of all persons. Although wants may also be of legitimate ethical concern, they must wait for later consideration, until needs are met. For example, when hospital beds are in short supply, the decision-making process that will allocate this resource must take into account the difference between an individual who needs a bed in order to be treated for a heart condition and a person who wants a bed to have cosmetic surgery. It could be argued that the psychological condition of a patient asking for cosmetic surgery moves this surgery into the "need" category, but the merits of this argument are only relative to the other competing needs. The questions that we must ask ourselves at this stage are: is the issue one of need or want? For whom is this a need? For whom is this a want?

Consult Legal and Ethical Guidelines

After we have clarified the nature of the issue, we must examine the relevant civil laws and/or ethics codes guidelines that are specific to the situation. The answers to the following questions will assist in this deliberation:

- What is the current legal opinion on this issue?
- Is there a reference to this issue in my own discipline's code of ethics? That of another discipline?

Examine Moral Responsibilities

The next step in this decision-making process is to consider our moral duties. These duties of beneficence, non-maleficence, justice, and honesty must all be examined in the context of the problem at hand. Consider the following questions:

- What is in the best interests of the patient?
- Will anyone be harmed by any possible solutions?
- Are all parties being given equivalent consideration? Are consistent criteria being used to determine this?
- Have I been honest with all involved parties?
- Is the truth being told or is something being held back?
- Am I being honest with myself about my thoughts and personal biases?

Uphold Patient Autonomy

Once our own moral duties have been considered, we have to ensure that patient autonomy is being taken into account and upheld to the extent that is possible. The individual's right to self-determination must be included in any discussion of an ethical problem in health care delivery. These questions will help to determine if this principle is being well considered:

- Have I given the patient (and/or family) enough information so that the principle of autonomy can be adequately carried out?
- What are the patient's (and/or family's) opinions?
- Are there any complicating problems, e.g. competency?

Evaluate Possible Solutions

As we come closer to the decision, we need to determine if the proposed solutions produce benefits or burdens. This issue of benefit vs. burden is very important in the solution of problems in health care ethics. The following questions assist to evaluate the extent of this concern:

- Can this solution easily be classified as a benefit or a burden? To whom?
- Are the benefits and burdens fairly distributed?

For example, the decision to withhold treatment from a seriously ill, deformed neonate must be evaluated in the context of its benefits and burdens. Would such a decision result in a benefit for the parents, who then would not have to prolong their grief and provide for a severely handicapped child, or would the decision create for them a burden of guilt in hastening the death of their infant? Is the decision of benefit to the child, by shortening the time spent in pain, or is it a burden because the child's chance of any kind of a life is destroyed?

Make the Decision

Finally, after considering all the preceding questions and all the possible solutions, what is our decision? Whenever a decision is made, indecision can still be present. Thus, when a solution to an ethical dilemma is finally agreed upon, but before it is implemented, we should apply some tests to determine if we have truly arrived at the right decision to the best of our abilities. As a final step in the decision-making process, examine your decision and ask yourself the following questions about it:

- What is your intention in making this decision?
- Would you be ready to discuss this decision with all affected parties before its implementation?
- Would you be happy to tell your mother/father/husband/wife/significant other that you had made such a decision?
- Would you be satisfied to have it publicly known that you made this kind of a decision?
- How would you view this decision if you sat on the other side of the fence?
- How do you expect this decision will be viewed by others?

These questions are designed to examine the extent to which you are being true to your own personal values. If you are dissatisfied with your own response to any of these questions, you can return to any step in the process and go through that process again with a different solution in mind. Thus, the final question that needs to be asked is: do I need to filter or review this decision again?

Some Caveats to Consider

One always proposes a framework for ethical decision making with some trepidation. First, there is the fear that health care workers, despite admonishments to the contrary, will use such a framework to provide themselves with a cookbook approach to finding solutions to complex moral problems. Second, using a framework like this can lead to the conclusion that *rule ethics* is a preferable approach to *situational ethics,* although in practice the framework allows a blending of both approaches. We caution the reader against any such conclusions.

Remember that the principles named in this or any other approach are best interpreted as checklists to ensure that all the relevant considerations have been taken into account. In addition, never forget that ethical principles, regardless of how frequently one finds them in ethics textbooks, have yet to be empirically justified. For example, apart from the writings of very erudite individuals and scholars from Hippocrates and Aristotle to modern medical ethicists, and notwithstanding the fact that they have been incorporated into modern codes of ethics, even principles such as beneficence and non-maleficence have yet to be empirically justified, nor is this likely ever to change. While we presume them to be correct, we are uncertain even as to how we might go about testing them.

Finally, in using a framework such as the one we have suggested, you need to be continually aware that you are applying a number of principles which may at times conflict. At the present time, there is no universal and unified theory of health care ethics. Thus, every time you must consider a number of ethical principles in the solution of one problem, there is a risk that those principles themselves will come into conflict with each other.

> An adequate ethical theory should not be just some more or less systematically related set of principles and rules. Rather it should provide an explanation of our moral agreement and disagreement; it should organize our moral thinking; it should tell us what is relevant to a moral judgement. (Clouser and Gert, 1990, p. 232)

Someday, perhaps, a unified moral theory will evolve. Until then, the percolation plan is presented as a framework for making practical decisions in health care settings.

Summary

To deal with health care ethics is no easy matter and will undoubtedly become even more difficult as medical technology advances. If we persist in regarding "medical ethics," "nursing ethics," "pharmacy ethics," "physiotherapy ethics," etc., as separate areas of consideration, the richness of interdisciplinary thought will be lost.

As workers in the delivery of health care, we need to work together to find a consistent approach that all members of all disciplines can use to identify moral behavior and to find the best solutions to ethical dilemmas.

Recommended Reading

Jonsen, A.R. "Of Balloons and Bicycles, or, The Relationship between Ethical Theory and Practical Judgement," *Hastings Center Report,* 21 (September-October, 1991), 14-16.

Appendices

Cases for Further Discussion

The following cases illustrate many of the issues presented in the preceding chapters. They may be useful for class discussion, examination questions, or as the basis for research papers designed to examine the issues more fully. In addition, practitioners may find them useful for clarification of their own values.

CASE 1: Defective Newborns

Susan F. is a 20-year-old unmarried woman who has just given birth to an infant who has been diagnosed as suffering from Down's Syndrome, complicated by a minor heart defect and an esophageal malformation. While the degree of mental retardation cannot be determined yet and the heart condition is not life-threatening, the esophageal problem is such that the child cannot have a normal intake of food and fluids and must receive intravenous fluids until surgery to repair the esophageal malformation. This operation, in the surgeon's opinion, ought to be done as soon as possible.

With no family or close friends, and no job, Susan is destitute. She had not wanted to carry the child to term, but refused to face the inevitability of her pregnancy until it was too far advanced to seek an abortion. Now, she has told the nurses that she cannot care for any child, let alone a defective one, and wishes that the child be left alone to die. To this end, she has refused to sign consent for the surgery, wishes food and fluids to be stopped, and has told the nurses that she will take the baby home with her against medical advice if any such measures are instituted.

The surgeon has acquiesced to the mother's wishes, but the nurses disagree and have informed him that they will seek a court injunction unless basic treatment of food and fluids is reinstituted.

CASE 2: Refusal of Treatment

Mrs. J. is a 54-year-old widow who was diagnosed with multiple sclerosis at the age of 40. Since that time, she has suffered progressive deterioration to the point where she is now confined to a wheelchair although she continues to maintain her independence, living in her own apartment where a nurse visits her every day. In the past five years, her vision has declined, and she has suffered from recurrent urinary tract infections, but her mental acuity continues to be normal.

She is now admitted to the hospital with bronchopneumonia, another condition that seems to be recurring, as this is the third bout in less than a year. The admitting physician has recommended antibiotic therapy, which Mrs. J. has refused up to this point. She is tired of being ill and has no desire to be what she calls a burden to her children any longer.

Her five grown children have never expressed the idea that she is a burden of any kind, and the three who live close by visit every day, bringing the three grandchildren whenever possible. They, however, are respectful of their mother's wishes and support her decision to refuse any further treatment.

Mrs. J.'s two remaining children, both of whom live halfway across the country, have telephoned the doctor and insist that treatment be initiated.

CASE 3: Do-Not-Resuscitate

Ms. L. is a 29-year-old woman who, seven weeks ago, fell from a fourth floor balcony while attempting to retrieve her cat and was admitted to the neurosurgical unit with severe head injuries that have resulted in a sustained coma. Twice in the first two weeks after her admission, and once in the sixth week, she suffered cardio-respiratory arrest and was successfully resuscitated. The neurosurgical team believes that her coma is irreversible and have informed her husband of this. When questioned about their certainty, the team members agreed that no one can ever be absolutely certain in these situations. The team has recommended to the husband that a do-not-resuscitate order be instituted, and he has refused.

The nurses on the unit are becoming increasingly concerned about the necessity to resuscitate Ms. L. and, when approached again, Mr. L. describes his hope that a miracle might occur for the sake of his wife and their two young children. He does, however, admit to being unable to face the decision.

CASE 4: AIDS

Mr. K. is a 45-year-old married man who has never frequented the doctor's office. One afternoon, he appears in the office of the physician who has treated his wife and two children for many years and asks to be screened for gonorrhea and syphilis. Upon further questioning by the physician, the patient reveals that he has been unfaithful to his wife and, in fact, has been engaging in bisexual relationships for the past decade. He has recently become concerned about STDs, because of their prominence in the media, and wishes to be screened in total privacy.

The doctor asks him if he wishes to be screened for HIV, and he refuses. The physician explains to him that should he test positive for these diseases, his wife, who is also at risk, needs to be told. He refuses to allow the physician to inform his wife, as his "other life" is a complete secret to her, and he wishes to keep it that way. His wife is currently pregnant with their third child.

CASE 5: Sex Preselection

Mr. and Mrs. H., both 40 years old, are the parents of three teenaged sons. With a comfortable life ahead of them, and their family completed, Mrs. H. finds, to her utter amazement, that she is pregnant. While neither of them really wants another child and both recognize the genetic risks inherent because of Mrs. H.'s age, she has always had an unspoken desire to have a daughter.

Thus, while not at all enthusiastic about the idea of having a fourth child, the couple are ambivalent and are tempted to continue the pregnancy to the point where a prenatal diagnosis might be possible. While Mrs. H.'s age makes amniocentesis advisable in this pregnancy anyway, their criteria for possible termination at that point would include the sex of the child. They would be willing to have a girl, but not another boy.

CASE 6: Religious Beliefs and Medical Decisions

Mrs. S., a 50-year-old widow, is rushed to the emergency room of the community hospital following a motor vehicle accident, suffering from internal bleeding, profuse external bleeding, and impending shock. The family physician on duty in the emergency room orders intravenous glucose, to be followed immediately by Ringer's Lactate.

While searching for the name of her next-of-kin in the patient's purse, a nurse discovers a card indicating that Mrs. S. is a Jehovah's Witness and that she is not to be given a blood transfusion under any circumstances. Although the card is signed, it is neither dated nor witnessed.

A search for family is made, but none is immediately available. The doctor determines that blood transfusions are necessary to save Mrs. S.'s life, administers them, and sends her on to surgery. The following day, the patient's son arrives and signs a form indicating that no blood or blood products are to be given to his mother under any circumstances. The doctor refuses to follow the instructions of the son.

Three weeks later, Mrs. S. is discharged home, having made a full recovery from her injuries. One month later, Mrs. S. files suit against the doctor and the hospital.

CASE 7: Patient Autonomy

Mr. A. is a 45-year-old man who presents himself at his doctor's office complaining of a runny nose, cough, and sore throat—symptoms compatible with an acute viral infection. The doctor advises the patient to go home, take it easy, and take an analgesic and a decongestant as necessary every four hours.

Mr. A. informs the doctor that the only reason he made this visit was to obtain a prescription for penicillin. The doctor explains to Mr. A. that a viral infection of this nature would not respond to penicillin and refuses to write the prescription. Mr. A. says that he has received penicillin for these symptoms on prior occasions and that it has resulted in full recovery, so he continues to demand it.

CASE 8: Conflicting Obligations

Mr. F. is a 40-year-old married man who is admitted to the intensive care unit following an acute myocardial infarct. He has suffered complete cardio-respiratory arrest at home before the ambulance arrived, and, although CPR was initiated immediately upon the arrival of the medics, the patient has been in full arrest for ten minutes and never regains consciousness.

The primary nurse caring for Mr. F. comes to know his wife and three children and sees how much they suffer as they watch modern medicine struggle to save his life. Ten days later, he finally dies.

The intern approaches Mrs. F. to request permission for an autopsy, and she refuses. She then refuses the resident, who tells her that she will be impeding medical science, but she maintains that she wishes her husband to have some small measure of dignity. Finally, the chief of the unit persuades her to consent. The nurse, who feels that she understands Mrs. F.'s refusal, thinks that perhaps she should have supported her in her decision, but at the same time recognizes that there is a legitimate need to perform autopsies.

CASE 9: Research Ethics

Mr. B. has been a pharmacist in the community hospital for the past ten years. During that time, he has noted that two of the urologists routinely prescribe the same medication for preoperative prophylaxis in their prostate surgery patients. A month ago, he noted that one of the doctors changed his prescribing routine; when questioned about the change, the doctor told Mr. B. that he and the other urologist wished to see if this new medication was as effective as the old one in preventing post-operative infections.

Mr. B. mentions this to the Director of Pharmacy, who checks to see if there has been a research protocol passed by the hospital's research ethics committee and if each patient had consented to being part of the trial. When no such proposal is found, the doctors are approached again, and they inform the pharmacists that because both drugs were commercially available no such protocol was necessary—that this is not a bona fide research project.

The Director of Pharmacy is uneasy about this explanation and, upon further investigation, finds that both of the urologists in question have recently attended an educational seminar in Boston, all expenses paid by the pharmaceutical manufacturer of the newer drug.

CASE 10: Consent

Mr. K. is a 70-year-old resident of the long-term wing of the hospital, who has been admitted because of his end-stage COPD. With a 24-hour-a-day requirement for oxygen, he is no longer able to care for himself at home and expects to live out his final months here in peace. His doctor has ordered that he receive a respiratory evaluation and an aide wheels him into the physical therapy department against his will.

When Mr. K. refuses the tests, the therapist begins to tell him about the benefits of obtaining baseline information on his admittance to this new facility to aid in possible future therapy. Mr. K. obviously does not want the tests, nor any further therapy. The therapist continues to cajole Mr. K., until he finally throws up his hands in disgust and tells him that he will submit to the tests if everyone will just leave him alone after that.

The Oath of Hippocrates

I swear by Apollo, the Physician, by Aesculapius, by Hygeia, by Panacea, by all the gods and goddesses, to keep according to my ability and my judgement, the following Oath:

"To hold the one who taught me this art equally precious to me as my parents; to share my assets with him and, if need be, to see to his needs; to treat his children in the same manner as my brothers and to teach them this art free of charge or stipulation, if they desire to learn it; that by maxim, lecture and every other method of teaching, I will bestow a knowledge of the art to my own sons, to the sons of my teacher and to disciples who are bound by a contract and oath, according to the law of medicine and to no one else; I will adhere to that method of treatment which, to the best of my ability and judgement, I consider beneficial for my patients and I will disavow whatever is harmful and illegal; I will administer no fatal medicine to anyone even if solicited, nor will I offer such advice; in addition, I will not provide a woman with an implement useful for abortion.

"I will live my life and practice my art with purity and reverence. I will not operate on someone who is suffering from a stone but will leave this to be done by those who perform such work. Whatever house I enter, I will go therein for the benefit of the sick and I will stand free from any voluntary criminal action and corrupt deed and the seduction of females or males, be they slaves or free. I will not divulge anything that, in connection with my profession or otherwise, I may see or hear of the lives of men which should not be revealed, on the belief that all such things should be kept secret.

"So long as I continue to be true to this Oath, may I be granted happiness of life, the practice of my art and the continuing respect of all men. But if I forswear and violate this Oath, may my fate be the opposite."

Patient Questionnaire on Advance Directives

Today families and physicians often face difficult decisions about life-prolonging procedures in case of terminal illness or severe accident. In such situations it is of great help to have some knowledge of how the patient when alert and competent viewed the issue of being maintained by machines.

The purpose of our discussion is to explore your desires in case of incapacitating illness. If you should become ill and your illness would make it impossible for you to communicate there would be a record of your wishes regarding treatment. It would be helpful if you would answer the questions on this paper. Thank you.

NAME _____ HOME PHONE _____

ADDRESS _____ CITY _____ STATE_____ ZIP _____

PERSON TO CONTACT IN CASE OF EMERGENCY _____PHONE NUMBER_____

                Relationship_____

PERSON YOU MOST TRUST WITH

YOUR PERSONAL DECISIONS_____PHONE NUMBER_____

                Relationship_____

IN GENERAL, DO YOU WISH TO PARTICIPATE OR SHARE IN MAKING DECISIONS ABOUT YOUR HEALTH CARE AND TREATMENT?   YES _____ NO _____

WOULD YOU ALWAYS WANT TO KNOW THE TRUTH ABOUT YOUR CONDITION?

                                                   YES _____ NO _____

ARE THERE ANY SPECIFIC RELIGIOUS OR OTHER WISHES YOU WOULD LIKE TO RECORD IN
REGARD TO YOUR HEALTH CARE?
(for instance prohibition of blood transfusion) _____

HAVE YOU SIGNED A LIVING WILL?   YES _____ NO _____

WOULD YOU BE INTERESTED IN A SAMPLE COPY OF A LIVING WILL? YES _____ NO _____

ARE YOU IN PRINCIPLE OPPOSED TO ORGAN DONATION?   YES _____ NO _____

WOULD YOU, IF THE OCCASION AROSE, WANT TO HAVE
YOUR ORGANS DONATED TO SOMEONE ELSE?   YES _____ NO _____

IN THE EVENT OF A SEVERE, ACUTE, OR CHRONIC ILLNESS WHICH LEAVES YOU MENTALLY
INCOMPETENT, WOULD YOU DESIRE TO BE KEPT ALIVE INDEFINITELY AT ALL COSTS?
                                                        YES _____ NO _____

HAVE YOU DISCUSSED YOUR FEELINGS ABOUT DEATH AND DYING WITH YOUR FAMILY?
          YES _____ NO _____ WITH WHOM? _____
                                       Relationship _____

IS THERE ANYONE ELSE WHO KNOWS YOUR WISHES REGARDING YOUR DEATH?
          NAME _____
          Relationship _____

WOULD YOU PREFER TO DIE AT HOME?   YES _____ NO _____
          IN THE HOSPITAL?   YES _____ NO _____
          NO PREFERENCE?   YES _____ NO _____

HOW WOULD YOU LIKE YOUR FUNERAL ARRANGED?
          BURIAL   YES _____ NO _____
          CREMATION   YES _____ NO _____

WHO WOULD BE IN CHARGE OF MAKING ARRANGEMENTS?
          NAME _____
          Relationship _____

AGE:_____ MARITAL STATUS: M__ S__ D__ W__   OCCUPATION: _____ SEX: _____
DATE:_____   SIGNATURE: _____
FURTHER COMMENTS:_____
_____

Sample Living Will

To My Family, My Physician, My Lawyer And All Others Whom It May Concern

Death is as much a reality as birth, growth, and aging—it is the one certainty in life. In anticipation of decisions that may have to be made about my own dying and as

an expression of my right to refuse treatment, I, _____, being of
(PRINT NAME)

sound mind, make this statement of my wishes and instructions concerning treatment.

By means of this document, which I intend to be legally binding, I direct my physician and other care providers, my family, and any surrogate designated by me or appointed by a court, to carry out my wishes. If I become unable, by reason of physical or mental incapacity to make decisions about my medical care, let this document provide the guidance and authority needed to make any and all such decisions.

If I am permanently unconscious or there is no reasonable expectation of my recovery from a seriously incapacitating or lethal illness or condition, I do not wish to be kept alive by artificial means. I request that I be given all care necessary to keep me comfortable and free of pain, even if pain-relieving medications may hasten my death, and I direct that no life-sustaining treatment be provided except as I or my surrogate specifically authorize.

This request may appear to place a heavy responsibility upon you, but by making this decision according to my strong convictions, I intend to ease that burden. I am acting after careful consideration and with understanding of the consequences of your carrying out my wishes.

List optional specific provisions in the space below.

Durable Power of Attorney for Health Care Decisions
(Cross out if you do not wish to use this section)

To effect my wishes, I designate _____, residing at

_____,

(phone #) _____, [or if he or she shall for any reason fail to

act, _____, residing at _____

_____, (phone #) _____]

as my health care surrogate—that is, my attorney-in-fact regarding any and all
health care decisions to be made for me, including the decision to refuse life-sustaining treatment—if I am unable to make such decisions myself. This power shall
remain effective during and not be affected by my subsequent illness, disability or
incapacity. My surrogate shall have authority to interpret my Living Will, and shall
make decisions about my health care as specified in my instructions or, when my
wishes are not clear, as the surrogate believes to be in my best interests. I release
and agree to hold harmless my health care surrogate from any and all claims
whatsoever arising from decisions made in good faith in the exercise of this power.

I sign this document knowingly, voluntarily, and after careful deliberation, this

_____ day of _____, 19____.

_____
(SIGNATURE)

Address _____

_____

WITNESS _____   WITNESS _____
PRINTED NAME _____   PRINTED NAME_____
ADDRESS _____   ADDRESS _____

_____   _____

I do hereby cerfity that the within document was executed and acknowledged before me by the principal this ____day of _____, 19___.

_____
NOTARY PUBLIC

Copies of this document have been given to:_____

_____

This Living Will expresses my personal treatment preferences. The fact that I may have also executed a declaration in the form recommended by state law should not be construed to limit or contradict this Living Will, which is an expression of my common-law and constitutional rights.

(Optional) My Living Will is registered with Concern for Dying (Registry No.____)

Reprinted by permission of Concern for Dying,
250 West 57th Street, New York, NY 10107
(212) 246-6962

References

"A Time to Die," *Canadian Medical Association Journal*, 142 (1990), 985-986.

Adler, M. *Ten Philosophical Mistakes*. New York: MacMillan Publishing Co., 1985.

"Alcoholics Get Low Priority for Liver Transplants," *Globe and Mail*, national ed., March 16, 1990, p. A10.

American Fertility Association, Ethics Committee of the... "Ethical Considerations of the New Reproductive Technologies," *Fertility and Sterility*, Supp. 1, 46 (September, 1986).

American Hospital Association. *Guidelines of Hospital Committees on Biomedical Ethics*. Chicago, 1983.

Annas, G. *The Rights of Patients: The Basic ACLU Guide to Patient Rights*. 2nd ed. Carbondale and Edwardsville: Southern Illinois University Press, 1989.

Aroskar, M.A. "Anatomy of an Ethical Dilemma: The Theory," *American Journal of Nursing*, 80 (April, 1980), 658-660.

Balkos, G. "The Ethically Trained Physician: Myth or Reality?" *Canadian Medical Association Journal*, 128 (March 15, 1983), 682-683.

Bandman, E.L. and B. Bandman. *Nursing Ethics Through the Lifespan*. 2nd ed. Norwalk, Conn.: Appleton and Lange, 1990.

Bayer, R. and others. "The Care of the Terminally Ill: Morality and Economics," *New England Journal of Medicine*, 309 (December 15, 1983), 1490-1494.

Beck, M. "The Geezer Boom," *Newsweek,* special issue, (Winter-Spring, 1990), 62-62, 66, 68.

Berger, J. H. and others. "Informed Consent: How Much Does the Patient Understand?" *Clinical Pharmacology and Therapeutics*, 27 (April, 1980), 435-439.

Buckman, R. and J. Senn. "Eligibility for CPR: is Every Death a Cardiac Arrest?" *Canadian Medical Association Journal*, 140 (May 1, 1989), 1068-1069.

Callahan, D. "Can We Return Death to Disease?" *Hastings Center Report*, Suppl., 19 (January-February, 1989), 4-6.

Callahan, D. *What Kind of Life.* New York: Simon and Shuster, 1990.

Canadian Medical Association. Code of Ethics. Ottawa, April, 1990.

Canadian Medical Protective Association. *Consent: A Guide for Canadian Physicians.*

Childress, J. "Triage in Neonatal Intensive Care: The Limitation of a Metaphor," *Virginia Law Review*, 69 (1983), 547-561.

Consumer Guide, ed. *Health Careers: Where the Jobs Are and How to Get Them.* New York: Fawcett Columbine, 1980.

Cresswell, S. "Doctor-Patient Communications: A Review of the Literature," *Ontario Medical Review*, (November, 1983), 559-556.

Crump, W.J. "Helping Your Patient Prepare a Living Will," *Senior Patient*, (March-April, 1989), 85-92.

Davies, J. "Raping and Making Love are Different Concepts: So Are Killing and Voluntary Euthanasia," *Journal of Medical Ethics*, 14 (September, 1988), 148-149.

deDombal, F.T. "Ethical Considerations Concerning Computers in Medicine in the 1980's," *Journal of Medical Ethics*, 13 (December, 1987), 179-184.

Dickey, N.W. "Physicians and Acquired Immunodeficiency Syndrome: A Reply to Patients," *Journal of the American Medical Association*, 262 (October 13, 1989), 2002.

Dorland's Illustrated Medical Dictionary. 24th ed. Philadelphia: W.B. Saunders, 1965.

Eisenberg, J.M. and A.J. Rosoff. "Physician Responsibility for the Cost of Unnecessary Medical Services," *New England Journal of Medicine*, 299 (July 13, 1978), 76-80.

Emson, H.E. "Confidentiality: A Modified Value," *Journal of Medical Ethics*, 14 (June, 1988), 87-91.

Fleetwood, J.E.; R.M. Arnold, and R.J. Baron. "Giving Answers or Raising Questions?: The Problematic Role of Institutional Ethics Committees," *Journal of Medical Ethics*, 15 (September, 1989), 137-142.

Fost, N. "Ethical Issues in the Treatment of Critically Ill Newborns," *Pediatric Annals*, 10 (October, 1981), 16-21.

Foster, T.S. and C.L. Raehl. "Legal and Ethical Issues in Clinical Pharmacy Research: Informed Consent, Part I," *Drug Intelligence and Clinical Pharmacy*, 14 (January, 1980), 41-43.

Fox, R. "Training in Caring Competence in North American Medicine," *Humane Medicine*, 6 (Winter, 1990), 15-21.

Fried, C. "An Analysis of 'Equality and Rights' in Medical Care," *Nursing Digest*, (Spring, 1977), 68-70.

Friedrich, O. "One Miracle, Many Doubts," *Time*, December 10, 1984, 42, 44, 57-58.

Gerbert, B. and others. "Physicians and Acquired Immunodeficiency Syndrome: What Patients Think About Human Immunodeficiency Virus in Medical Practice," *Journal of the American Medical Association*, 262 (October 13, 1989), 1969-1972.

Gibbs, N. "Sick and Tired," *Time*, July 31, 1989, 28-33.

Gilmore, A. "Sanctity of Life versus Quality of Life—The Continuing Debate," *Canadian Medical Association Journal*, 130 (January 13, 1984), 180-181.

_____. "The Nature of Informed Consent," *Canadian Medical Association Journal*, 132 (May 15, 1985), 1198-1203.

Gilmore, N. and M.A. Somerville. *Physicians, Ethics and AIDS*. Ottawa: The Canadian Medical Association, 1989.

Grady, C. "Ethical Issues in Providing Nursing Care to Human Immunodeficiency Virus-Inflicted Populations," *Nursing Clinics of North America*, 24 (June, 1989), 523-534.

Greaves, D. "The Future Prospect for Living Wills," *Journal of Medical Ethics*, 15 (December, 1984), 179-182.

Haslam, R. "Rights of the Handicapped or Defective Infant," *Canadian Pediatric Society News Bulletin Supplement*, X (October-November, 1979), 1-4.

"Health Care Costs Set US Record," *Halifax Herald*, December 27, 1990, p. A19.

Herbert, V. "Acquiring New Information While Retaining Old Ethics," *Science*, 198 (November 18, 1977), 690-693.

Heussner, R.C. and M.E. Salmon. *Warning: The Media May be Harmful to Your Health*. Kansas City: Andrews and McMeel, 1988.

Higgins, G.L. "The History of Confidentiality in Medicine: The Physician-Patient Relationship," *Canadian Family Physician*, 35 (April, 1989), 921-926.

Hill, E. "Your Morality or Mine? An Inquiry into the Ethics of Human Reproduction—Presidential Address," *American Journal of Obstetrics and Gynecology*, 154 (June, 1986), 1173-1180.

Houlihan, P. *Life Without End: The Transplant Story*. Toronto: NC Press, 1988.

Hutchison, R. "The 'High-Tech Chronic': A New Kind of Patient," *Humane Medicine*, 4 (November, 1988), 118-119.

Infant Bioethics Task Force and Consultants. "Guidelines for Infant Bioethics Committees," *Pediatrics*, 74 (August, 1984), 306-311.

Inlander, C., L. Levin and E. Weiner. *Medicine on Trial*. New York: Prentice-Hall Press, 1988.

James, A., R. Zaner, J. Chapman, and C. Partain. "Technology and Turf: Medicine in Conflict," *Humane Medicine*, 6 (Autumn, 1990), 264-268.

Jankowic, E. *Behave Yourself*. Toronto: Prentice-Hall Canada, Inc., 1986.

Johnsen, D. "A New Threat to Pregnant Women's Autonomy," *Hastings Center Report*, 17 (August, 1987), 33-40.

Kapp, M.B. "Advance Health Care Planning: Taking a 'Medical Future'," *Southern Medical Journal*, 81 (1988), 221-224.

Kitzhauer, J. *The Oregon Basic Health Services Act*. Salem, Oregon: Legislative Assembly, 1989.

Kopelman, L. "Estimating Risk in Human Research," *Clinical Research*, 29 (February, 1981), 1-8.

Kutner, N. "Issues in the Application of High Cost Medical Technology: The Case of Organ Transplantation," *Journal of Health and Social Behavior*, 28 (March, 1987), 23-36.

Kuznar, N. "When It's Time to Die: Survey Reveals Physicians' Struggle with Ethics," *Modern Medicine,* 59 (July, 1991) 18, 20.

Leaf, A. "The Doctor's Dilemma—And Society's Too," *New England Journal of Medicine*, 310 (March 15, 1984), 718-721.

Lo, B. and S. Schroeder. "Frequency of Ethical Dilemmas in a Medical Inpatient Service," *Archives of Internal Medicine*, 141 (1981), 1062-1064.

Lyon, J. "Organ Transplants: Conundra Without End," *Second Opinion*, 1 (1987), 41-64.

Manuel, C. and others. "The Ethical Approach to AIDS: A Bibliographic Review," *Journal of Medical Ethics*, 16 (March, 1990), 14-27.

"Medical Confidentiality," *Briefings in Medical Ethics*, 16 (1990), 1-4.

Medical Research Council of Canada. Discussion Draft of Revised Guidelines on Research Involving Human Subjects, October, 1986, Ottawa, Canada.

"Medical Students Fear AIDS—Survey," *Halifax Herald*, Monday, May 21, 1990.

Moreno, J. "Ethics by Committee: The Moral Authority of Consensus," *Journal of Medicine and Philosophy*, 13 (November, 1988), 411-432.

Munday, T. Letter, *New England Journal of Medicine*, 323 (July 19, 1990), 201.

Newsom, D.; A. Scott, and J. Turk. *This is Public Relations*. Belmont, California: Wadsworth Publishing, 1987.

O'Neill, J. "Save Lives of Babies With Defects, MD's Told," *Toronto Globe and Mail*, Wednesday, November 30, 1983.

Parachini, A. "The California Humane and Dignified Death Initiative," *Hastings Center Report*, suppl., 19 (January-February, 1989), 10-12.

Parsons, A. "Allocating Health Care Resources: A Moral Dilemma," *Canadian Medical Association Journal*, 132 (February 15, 1985), 466-469.

Rachlis, M. and C. Kushner. *Second Opinion: What's Wrong with Canada's Health Care System and How to Fix It*. Toronto: Collins Pub., 1989.

Rauchman, S. and A. Tan. "Expediting the Transfer of Life," *Canadian Doctor*, 53 (May, 1987), 1, 4-8.

Rich, P. "Overtreating the Elderly Boosting Health Care Costs," *The Medical Post*, May 29, 1990, 22.

Robinson, G. and A. Merov. "Informed Consent: Recall by Patients Tested Postoperatively," *Annals of Thoracic Surgery*, 22 (September, 1976), 209-212.

Rooks, J. "Let's Admit We Ration Health Care—Then Set Priorities," *American Journal of Nursing*, 90 (June, 1990), 39-43.

Rothschild, J. "Engineering 'The Perfect Child': Toward a New Hierarchy of Birth," presentation at Mount Saint Vincent University, Halifax, Nova Scotia, January 17, 1991.

Rutter, P. *Sex in the Forbidden Zone*. Los Angeles: Jeremy P. Tarcher, Inc., 1986.

Sawyer, L. "Nursing Codes of Ethics: An International Comparison," *International Nursing Review*, 36 (September-October, 1989), 145-148.

Schafer, A. "Are Hospital Ethicists Doing a Worthwhile Job?" *Toronto Globe and Mail*, December 9, 1986, A7.

Schattschneider, H. "Power Relationships Between Physician and Nurse," *Humane Medicine*, 6 (Summer, 1990), 197-201.

Schiff, D. "Trouble Ahead: Decision-Making Concerns in Neonatology," *The Bioethics Bulletin*, 2 (December, 1990), 1-2.

Seiden, D. "Diminishing Choices, Critical Choices," *Commonwealth*, (March 8, 1985), 137-141.

Shorter, E. *Bedside Manners: The Troubled History of Doctors and Patients*. New York: Simon and Schuster, 1985.

_____. *The Health Century*. New York: Doubleday, 1987.

Silverman, W. "The Myth of Informed Consent: In Daily Practice and in Clinical Trials," *Journal of Medical Ethics*, 15 (March, 1989), 6-11.

Silversides, A. "Oregon Tackles the Health Care Rationing Issue," *Canadian Medical Association Journal*, 143 (September 15, 1990), 545-546.

Singer, P. "The Case of Nancy Cruzan, the Patient Self-Determination Act and Advance Directives in Canada," *Humane Medicine,* 7 (August, 1991), 225-227.

Sipes-Metzler, P. "Oregon Update," *Hastings Center Report* (September-October, 1991), 13.

Stein, L; D. Watts, and T. Howell. "The Doctor-Nurse Game Revisited," *New England Journal of Medicine*, 322 (February 22, 1990), 546-549.

Sullivan, P. "CMA's Discussion Paper on Fetal Rights May Spark Debate," *Canadian Medical Association Journal*, 143 (1990), 404-405.

Taylor, P. and R. Mickleburgh. "Dentists Strive to Calm Patients' Fears of AIDS," *The Globe and Mail*, April 17, 1991.

Veatch, R. "Medical Ethics," *Journal of the American Medical Association*, 252 (October 26, 1984), 2296-2300.

_____. "DRG's and the Ethical Reallocation of Resources," *Hastings Center Report*, (June, 1986), 32-40.

Wallis, C. "The New Origins of Life," *Time*, (September 10, 1984), 40, 42-44, 49, 51.

Washington Post Writer's Group. *Messages: The Washington Post Media Companion*. Boston: Allyn and Bacon, 1991.

Wertz, D. and J. Fletcher. "Fatal Knowledge? Prenatal Diagnosis and Sex Selection," *Hastings Centre Report*, 19 (May-June, 1989), 21-27.

Wiseman, H. "Ethical Choices in the Age of Pervasive Technology," *Westminster Affairs*, 3 (Fall, 1989), 3.

Wood, C. "The Transplant Revolution," *Macleans*, (November 23, 1987), 34-36, 38, 40.

Zilz, D. "Interdependence in Pharmacy: Risks, Rewards and Responsibilities," *American Journal of Hospital Pharmacy*, 47 (August, 1990), 1759-1765.

Glossary

agapism   to show loving concern; love for mankind.

autonomy   respecting a person's right to self-determination.

beneficence   the principle of "doing good."

consequentalist   see "utilitarianism."

deontological   the moral theories that are based on the concept of inalienable rights that must be respected and protected with little reference to consequences; duty-based.

ethimetrics   the application of amount and probability statistics to macro-moral problems of distributive justice.

eugenics   the science of improving the physical and mental qualities of the human race through control of the factors that influence heredity.

euthanasia   deliberate intervention to bring about the death of another human being where the intent is to do good; an easy death.

iatrogenesis   illness resulting from treatment modalities.

non-maleficence   the principle of "doing no harm."

normative ethics   dealing with norms of obligations and norms of values.

paternalism   making decisions for patients based on the belief that the caregiver knows what is best.

pluralism   a condition of society in which disparate religious, ethnic, and racial groups are part of a common community.

pragmatism   the notion that ideas and decisons are valuable only in terms of their practical consequences; outcomes are the test of the validity or truth of one's beliefs.

teleological   the moral theories that are based on the concept of outcomes.

thanatology   the study of death and dying.

utilitarianism   decision making based on the belief that ends justify means.

Index